D0202070

Healthcare Outcomes Management: Strategies for Planning and Evaluation

Dale J. Block, MD, CPE

Assistant Professor
Department of Health Management Systems
Duquesne University
Rangos School of Health Sciences
Pittsburgh, Pennsylvania

Medical Director/Family physician
Greentree Medical Associates
Allegheny Medical Practice Network
West Penn Allegheny Health System
Pittsburgh, Pennsylvania

JONES AND BARTLETT PUBLISHERS
Sudbury, Massachusetts
BOSTON   TORONTO   LONDON   SINGAPORE

World Headquarters

Jones and Bartlett Publishers	Jones and Bartlett Publishers	Jones and Bartlett Publishers
40 Tall Pine Drive	Canada	International
Sudbury, MA 01776	6339 Ormindale Way	Barb House, Barb Mews
978-443-5000	Mississauga, Ontario L5V 1J2	London W6 7PA
info@jbpub.com	CANADA	UK
www.jbpub.com		

Jones and Bartlett's books and products are available through most bookstores and online book-sellers. To contact Jones and Bartlett Publishers directly, call 800-832-0034, fax 978-443-8000, or visit our website www.jbpub.com.

Substantial discounts on bulk quantities of Jones and Bartlett's publications are available to corporations, professional associations, and other qualified organizations. For details and specific discount information, contact the special sales department at Jones and Bartlett via the above contact information or send an email to specialsales@jbpub.com.

Library of Congress Cataloging-in-Publication Data
Block, Dale J.
   Healthcare outcomes management : strategies for planning and
evaluation / Dale J. Block.
      p. cm.
   Includes bibliographical references and index.
   ISBN-10: 0-7637-3389-X (pbk.)
   1. Outcome assessment (Medical care) 2. Medical care--Quality
control. 3. Medical care--Evaluation.   I. Title.
   [DNLM: 1. Outcome Assessment (Health Care)--methods.
   2. Outcome Assessment (Health Care)--organization & administration.
   3. Delivery of Health Care--methods. 4. Delivery of Health Care
   --organization & administration.   W 84.1 B651h 2006]
   R853.O87B56 2006
   362.1068--dc22

                                        2005027422
   6048   ISBN-13: 978-0-7637-3389-6

Production Credits
Publisher: Michael Brown
Production Director: Amy Rose
Production Editor: Tracey Chapman
Associate Editor: Kylah Goodfellow McNeill
Associate Marketing Manager: Marissa Hederson
Manufacturing and Inventory Coordinator: Amy Bacus
Composition: Arlene Apone
Cover Design: Timothy Dziewit
Printing and Binding: Malloy, Inc.
Cover Printing: Malloy, Inc.

Printed in the United States of America
10 09 08 07 06   10 9 8 7 6 5 4 3 2 1

Dedication

This book is dedicated to the memories of my daughter, Julie Ann Block, and my great-niece, Eliana Sweatland, who were taken from our midst without having the opportunity to live a full and productive life on this Earth. This book is also dedicated to my wife, Ellen, and my three sons; Aaron, Jeremy, and Stuart, who have supported my efforts to formalize the many ideas that we have discussed over the years regarding healthcare delivery and outcomes management and planning.

Table of Contents

Preface

The 20th century experienced a great healthcare revolution. New medical treatments and the exponential growth of healthcare facilities and practitioners led the way to an abundance of healthcare goods and services. The efficacy, effectiveness, efficiency, humanity, and equity in the delivery of healthcare goods and services have historically relied on the intuition and subjective assessments of health professionals who used personal experience and clinical anecdotes to evaluate performance. Over time, a movement to a more scientific and systematic approach to healthcare outcomes management and planning took center stage for a number of reasons. The latter part of the 20th century noted shifts toward patients' rights and a consumerist model of healthcare delivery. Medical errors in diagnosis and treatment resulted in higher than normal rates of morbidity and mortality, escalated healthcare inflation rates, and lowered patient satisfaction with healthcare delivery systems.

There are two main models of healthcare delivery that serve as the framework for understanding healthcare outcomes management and planning today. The first healthcare delivery model is the "biomedical approach" to patient care. Established as the main model of healthcare delivery during the 20th century, the biomedical approach has its roots in the 1600s, when the great scientific thinkers of that time began to question how science and scientific inquiry could better answer the questions surrounding the problems of the human body. Based upon years of study of the human body—from the organ level to the micromolecular level—there are five doctrines that make up the biomedical approach to patient care: mind-body dualism, the mechanical analogy, physical reductionism, specific etiology, and reduction and control. These doctrines enable the clinician and the healthcare delivery system to focus only on the individual disease state and to reduce it to its most basic form of structural alteration or physiologic malfunction for diagnosis and treatment. Clinical outcomes, including morbidity and mortality, have been the mainstay of healthcare outcomes management. This system uses only the biomedical approach to patient care, and has little concern for the patient as a whole being. Biological issues that may result from psychological and social pressures to influence the patient's health and well-being are not considered.

The other healthcare delivery model is the "biopsychosocial approach" to patient care. This model serves as an integrated approach to managing patients within the healthcare delivery system. It is also based on principles of science and scientific inquiry. However, the biopsychosocial approach differs from the biomedical approach in the way patients are viewed by clinicians at the point of care. The biopsychosocial approach examines and evaluates the patient with a combined view of individual and population health, illness, and disease. At the point of care, the biopsychosocial approach elicits the patient's story and life circumstances; integrates the biological, psychological, social, and environmental domains; recognizes the centrality of relationships in providing health care to patients and populations; understands the healthcare practitioner; focuses the model for clinical practice based on population-based medicine; and provides multidimensional treatments based on evidenced-based medicine.

Healthcare Outcomes Management explores the critical assessment of healthcare outcomes management and planning using the biopsychosocial approach of healthcare delivery as the framework for discussion. In this discussion, the following assumptions are accepted about the American healthcare delivery system: there is a limit to the resources that can be made available for healthcare delivery; an effort must be made to match the healthcare service needs of the population to the healthcare goods and services that are allocated within the delivery system; because healthcare inflation is rising, it is necessary to choose those healthcare interventions that produce the greatest health gains at the lowest cost to the greatest number of people; and historical patterns of supply and demand have influenced the type and location of health care currently provided.

Current prominent texts that explore healthcare outcomes management and planning use the biomedical model as their framework for discussion. In today's tumultuous times in healthcare delivery, the biopsychosocial model is more complete and addresses both the changes in patient's rights and the swing to a consumerist model of healthcare delivery.

Healthcare Outcomes Management will enable the reader to develop a thorough understanding of the biopsychosocial model of healthcare delivery and its relevance to the systematic evaluation of healthcare interventions. This book focuses on the processes of healthcare evaluation that seeks to analyze healthcare interventions available to healthcare consumers in terms of four principle dimensions: effectiveness, efficiency, humanity, and equity. These principles help guide the formal, systematic evaluation process that determines the greatest benefit for healthcare consumers with the least amount of risk for adverse outcomes. Careful attention to the basic principles of epidemiology, healthcare economics, medical ethics, population medicine, medical informatics, and environmental health have also been included in the book to increase the reader's appreciation for the applied medical sciences and their applications to the delivery of healthcare services at the point of care.

This book also includes a number of different measuring methodologies, and their strengths and weaknesses as they apply to healthcare outcomes management and planning. In today's economic times, the saying goes: "No measure, no margin; no margin, no mission!" American healthcare consumers today are searching for value and quality at the point of care because of the cost-shifting that has occurred as a result of double digit healthcare inflation. Now more than ever, with an aging population and an increasing reliance on technology, patients and clinicians need to partner together to have a better understanding of which healthcare interventions will enhance the patient's overall health, functionality, and quality of life.

It is my hope that this book will provide the many necessary tools used in the biopsychosocial approach to healthcare outcomes management and planning for those who have accepted the role of providing healthcare resources, both clinically and administratively, to patients at the point of care.

Dale J. Block, MD, CPE

CHAPTER 1

Introduction to Healthcare Outcomes Management and Planning

HISTORY OF QUALITY MANAGEMENT— A STARTING POINT

Berwick, Godfrey, and Roessner provide an excellent short synopsis on the history of quality management (1990) which can be summarized as follows. Quality management began as a very simple activity. Craftsmen were known to inspect their work during production and at the completion of their project. Apprentices, who were learning the craft, had their work approved before starting a project and inspected both during the production process and at the completion of the project. Over time, craftsmen (small business owners) were organized into larger production shops and factories, mainly for economic reasons. As craftsmen were reorganized, production became standardized and direct supervision of activities was no longer practical. A separate function was created to have work inspected on the shop floor. Inspectors were often craftsmen who were trained in the formal process of studying the outcomes of work. Inspectors decided how many samples to inspect from a lot and when to pass or discard the entire lot based on the results from the initial sample. Inspection as a separate function added cost to production; however it became an acceptable and necessary activity to protect consumers from receiving and using defective products.

Product inspection on the shop floor as a separate function was challenged by Walter Shewhart in the 1930s (Berwick, Godfrey, and Roessner, 1990, 30). His landmark book, *The Economic Control of Quality of Manufactured Product*, written in 1931, shifted the major industrial philosophical approach from finding and fixing problems in the *products of work* to finding and fixing problems in the *processes of work*. Shewhart believed that proper control of the processes of production were far more efficient than endpoint inspection to assure and improve quality.

Great Britain and the United States accepted this change in philosophy during the World War II era by adopting Shewhart's quality control methods. Post-World War II, his methodology was fully implemented in Japan, as this country began to rebuild its economy after the war. American experts, W. Edwards Deming and Joseph M. Juran, were sent—at United States government expense—to teach the Japanese Shewhart's model of quality control. The Japanese learned to apply these methods of quality control and improvement to all the business functions of a company: manufacturing, design, marketing distribution, sales, and service. Between 1950 and 1975, Americans learned little about quality management while Japan not only learned about quality management; they excelled at it, becoming experts in the field.

What did the Japanese learn about quality management that allowed them to rebuild their post-World War II economy into a world economic power? First, quality improvement guided by theory and systematic information can help complex systems of production to function at levels of quality, efficiency, productivity, and morale that usually cannot even be imagined in systems manipulated by misguided intuition and habitual forms of control. Second, systematic improvement of quality is both an art and a science, a managerial science guided by theories in statistics, engineering, psychology, and experience. Third, experimentation belongs on the shop floor. The greatest assets of any complex system are the people working in the system. With proper guidance and mentoring, the human thinkers and doers can convey their ideas of improvement into action. Fourth, managing quality is an exercise in enabling, not controlling. Defects in production result from a problem with the production process, not from the workers performing the tasks. Fifth, actions of managers to improve quality without proper education in the theory of quality management, called "tampering", can result in the demise of the production process with fear and waste overtaking the production workforce. Sixth, controlling the processes of production can lead to predictable processes of production. In quality, this means a more favorable production outcome and improvement in all facets of a company's bottom line. Quality control becomes a continuous search for small, incremental opportunities to reduce waste, rework, and unnecessary complexity.

American industry continued to turn a deaf ear upon the pursuits of quality management during the 1980s. In 1983, A. V. Feigenbaum updated his now famous book, *Total Quality Control,* first published in 1951, which emphasizes the importance of involving the entire corporate structure in quality management (Feigenbaum, 31). Feigenbaum's theory proposed total quality control as a system for integrating quality-related efforts throughout an organization so that all business functions could focus together on the efficient satisfaction of the customer's needs. The Japanese expounded on Feigenbaum's concepts to include participation of the entire work force in quality management regardless of hierarchical level. Company-wide total quality control involved a complete mobilization of improvement and control efforts—including all levels and all business functions—into one organizational effort.

Unfortunately for the American economy, many American companies collapsed under the brutal competition for national and international market share in the late 1980s and early 1990s. Because they failed to recognize the emerging competition in quality based on improving customer satisfaction and reducing costs of poor quality, American companies were unable to compete with those international companies who had been fine tuning their efforts in quality management.

That American industry has failed to recognize the theories and systematic approach to quality management also correlates with the demise of our American healthcare delivery system. The central theory behind quality management is that the processes, not the people, drive the quality movement in an organization. In health care, it has been long accepted that quality is a function of the physicians and other clinical providers of medical goods and services. Health care, for the last several decades has believed that when the physicians do their work properly, patients will benefit and healthcare delivery will be successful. Education and training of physicians during the twentieth century perpetuated this myth, and the general public as patients believed the same. Health care was not seen as a production process. So, when problems arise in healthcare delivery, people are blamed, and higher costs and poorer quality of care result.

BASIC PRINCIPLES OF QUALITY MANAGEMENT

Again, Berwick, Godfrey, and Roessner provide an excellent discourse on the basic tenets of Quality Management (1990). The following is a synopsis of their review. Modern quality management focuses on the production process, and can be applied to virtually any process of production. The theory explains terms that describe the components and processes of production, gives insight into the nature of quality and the causes of its failures, and discusses methods of planning, improving, and controlling quality. It is this explanation of the theory of quality management that enables all processes of production to be understood, and allows any organization, large or small, producing any kinds of goods and services, to improve.

Productive work is accomplished through processes. Each person in an organization is involved in one or more of the processes of production. The employee receives the work of others, adds value to the work received, and supplies it to the next employee in the production process. The employee (production worker) has a triple role: customer, processor, and supplier. As customers, employees receive various kinds of inputs from others to perform work essential to the production process. As processors, employees perform various managerial, technical, or administrative tasks in a sequence of steps using the inputs received. As suppliers, employees act as suppliers to other customers by delivering goods and/or services. By understanding the needs of the employee using this "triple role" concept (Berwick, Godfrey, and Roessner, 1990, 32), the quality of the production process can be improved at all points in the production process. This is a value-added endeavor for the ultimate customer who depends on the goods and services being produced. Health care has its own production processes each with its own customers and suppliers:

- Patient flow processes move patients from place to place in a hospital setting or within a healthcare delivery system
- Information flow processes create and transport data and information to allow for informed decisions to be made
- Material flow processes move equipment and supplies from place to place.

Quality management must see the world of production in terms of process no matter where the production process is found.

Sound customer-supplier relationships are absolutely necessary for sound quality management. Modern quality management is customer-focused. Improving the capability and reliability of the production process results in market share gain, higher prices in accord with higher value of the goods and/or services produced, and increased efficiency in production processes.

Customers are both internal and external to the production process. Quality management defines the customer as anyone who depends on the production process. Manufacturing companies have many customers such as direct purchasers, the community at large, secondary users of the company's goods and/or services, and the employees of the company. In healthcare delivery, the customers of the production process are many. Table 1-1 lists the major stakeholders affected by the healthcare delivery system.

Quality management maintains that good customer-supplier relationships—characterized by long-term commitments, clear communications, and mutual trust—are more likely to improve quality. It is a central concept in quality management that the quality of goods and/or services provided to external customers (between a company and its customers) is largely determined by the quality of goods and/or services exchanged between internal customers (those that lie within the production process) of the company. Modern quality management requires a great deal of

---

Table 1-1   Stakeholders in Healthcare Delivery

Consumers/Patients
Family and friends of patients
Community at large
Clinical providers of health care
Government
Health system administrators
Pharmaceutical companies
Pharmaceutical benefit management companies
Technology companies
Health plans
Private payers
Employers
Media representatives
Health services researchers
Academia

interaction, measurement, and clarification of roles that can help internal customers and suppliers understand and serve each other more effectively. The bottom line is the better the organization can understand and meet the needs of its diverse customers, the more successful it will be in the long run.

Because there are many complexities in the production process, the main source of quality defects is problems in the process. In fact, the complexities of the input/output subprocesses are many. These complexities result from the production processes evolving over time without a formal planning, documenting, implementing, and evaluating procedure. Emphasizing the importance of the production process is critical to overcome the many fundamental flaws that naturally occur as the production process becomes operational. It is the production process itself that creates the flaws, not the people. Hence, it follows that managers must exercise the authority, security, and autonomy to responsibly evaluate and change the production process to increase quality; they must not exhort and discipline the workers for flaws in the goods and/or services. The job of management, through monitoring, control, and incentive, is to lead the workers and mobilize their talents to ensure that he/she is functioning at the optimum level to work properly.

Poor quality is costly. Modern quality management seeks two types of quality improvement: improvements in quality that result from reduction in deficiencies and improvements that involve adding features to please or to meet the customer's needs. Freedom from deficiencies almost always reduces costs. New features to meet customer's needs may have advantages for an organization in gaining market share, enabling premium pricing, and increasing customer satisfaction and loyalty, which often initially results in an increase in production costs. However, this second improvement ultimately results in a net profit to the organization over time. Freedom from deficiencies can result in an overall savings to an organization by 25 to 30 percent of the total cost of production (Berwick, Godfrey, and Roessner, 1990, 38).

Careful attention to the design and control of the process prevents failures in the production process. The goal of quality control is to prevent defects before they must be repaired and to develop and maintain processes so reliable that inspection of the end result can be safely reduced or eliminated altogether. Relying on endpoint inspection to achieve quality is costly and inevitably imperfect. It is better to inspect and understand the operational characteristics of the production process so as to discover the ways in which flaws are introduced into goods and/or services.

Understanding the variability of processes is key to improving quality. In every process and in every measurement, variability exists. Health care recognizes this more than any type of production process. Understanding variation is key to gaining knowledge about performance. Today, it is possible to design a production process to function properly even in the face of variability. Identifying and controlling the sources of variation is critical to the production process—knowledge, skill, training, communication, and empowerment.

Quality control should focus on the most vital processes. The identification of the most important types and components of the production process results in an efficient quality management process. To assure the quality of each critical parameter of a process, managerial oversight must develop a clear definition of the desired quality performance level, a way to measure the performance, a way to interpret the measurements, and a way to take action to reestablish control when the production process is out of control. These are the basic elements of effective quality control.

The modern approach to quality is thoroughly grounded in scientific and statistical thinking. Scientific methodology holds the key to the improvement of the production process. In medicine, patients seek an explanation for symptoms, clinicians query and examine for signs of disease, diagnostic testing identifies and confirms the etiology of the disease process, patients and doctors agree on a treatment plan, and doctors assess the results of treatment to resolve the symptoms in the patient. It is this methodology that is scientific in its approach to the patient care process: perform diagnostic tests, formulate specific hypotheses of cause, test those hypotheses, design and apply remedies, and assess the effect of the remedies.

The scientific approach to quality is by its nature based on data. It is characteristic of quality management to invest resources and time in the design and implementation of measurement. Measurement is an extensive process that includes the measurement of customer's needs, supplier inputs to the production process, production process characteristics, and production results. These measures are used to gain knowledge of the production process so that they can be understood, predicted, and improved. Measurement is used so that everyone can control and improve processes, not so that some people can control other people. Modern health services research has identified and designed ways to measure and represent scientific concepts of physical function, emotional well-being, patient satisfaction, and activities of daily living, all outcomes of the healthcare delivery production process.

Total employee involvement is critical. The concept of supplier-processor-customer relationships (the "triple role") and the need for numerous controls and measurements throughout the organization make clear why everyone should be involved in quality control. Development of new organizational structures provides training for all employees in basic methodology for identifying problems or opportunities, for discovering causes, for developing and implementing remedies, and for establishing controls at the new levels.

New organizational structures can help achieve quality improvement. All organizations have had to develop new forms of management to accelerate quality improvement. Steering committees, quality councils, and project teams are required to give the quality improvement effort in an organization the ability and flexibility to provide structure, authority, security, and autonomy to make the preventive changes in the production processes resulting in high quality goods and /or services.

Quality management employs three basic, closely interrelated activities: quality planning, quality control, and quality improvement. *Quality planning* involves defining quality as it applies to customers, developing measures of quality, designing goods and/or services in accord with customer needs, designing processes capable of providing those goods and/or services, and transferring those processes into the routine operations of the organization. *Quality control* involves developing and maintaining operational methods to assure that processes work as they are designed to work and that target levels of performance are being achieved. Quality control requires a clear definition of quality; knowledge of expected performance; measurements of actual performance; a way to compare expected results to actual performance; and a way to take action when measured results are not equal to expected results, or when processes appear to be drifting from their expected performance levels. *Quality improvement* is the effort to improve the level of performance of a critical production process. It involves measuring the level of current performance, finding ways to improve that performance, and implementing new and better methods. Quality improvement is often where organizations begin in developing quality management programs.

No organization is perfect. However, the combination of statistical and scientific thinking, customer orientation, teamwork, total organizational involvement, clarity of mission, pride, continuous improvement, and profitability is found increasingly often among organizations that have learned how to manage and improve the quality of the goods and/or services produced in their organization.

CHAPTER 2

Quality Improvement in Health Care— Donabedian's Principles of Quality Improvement

INTRODUCTION TO DONABEDIAN'S PRINCIPLES OF QUALITY IMPROVEMENT

Avedis Donabedian's name is synonymous with quality of medical care. He is best known for his groundbreaking work in healthcare delivery which clearly defined the operational terms and the detailed blueprints for both its measurement, known as *quality assessment*, and its improvement, known as *quality assurance*. Donabedian demonstrated that quality in health care is an attribute of a system that he called *structure*, a set of organized activities that he called *process*, and an *outcome* that results from both. His last work (Donabedian, 2003) before he died, compiled his years of work into a concise, somewhat autobiographical story of quality assessment and assurance in simple, clear terms. Donabedian states in the introduction of his last book that he did not provide an exhaustive review on quality in health care, rather he provided "a personal statement of my own views and conclusions." The following is a synopsis of Donabedian's work, including the meaning of quality, its components, and Donabedian's clear and systematic guide to its assessment and enhancement in healthcare delivery. One cannot do justice to the healthcare outcomes measurement without first delving into the basics of quality in healthcare delivery interpreted from Donabedian's perspective.

THE MEANING OF QUALITY ASSURANCE

Donabedian defined quality assurance to mean "all actions taken to establish, protect, promote and improve the quality of health care." (Donabedian, 2003, XXIII) It was Donabedian's opinion that one cannot guarantee or assure quality. The goal is to increase the probability that the health care delivered will be good or better quality. Because there is no assurance that quality in health care is a given, Donabedian suggested *continuous improvement* (Donabedian, 2003, XXIV) to describe the quality in health care that is allusive and requires all to do better, eventually progressing to higher levels of goodness. *Quality management* (Donabedian, 2003, XXIV) in health care can also be used as a term to describe quality because it denotes a need for managerial oversight to ensure quality delivery of health care. As a means of familiarity and ease of use, Donabedian preferred *quality assurance* to describe quality in health care and thus the following discussion will also use this term.

TARGETS OF QUALITY ASSURANCE

The targets of quality assurance are the functions and activities that are subject to quality assurance. In health care, the targets of quality have traditionally been the services that clinicians provide directly to the patients. More recently, these targets have further expanded to include the functions and activities provided by all members of the healthcare delivery team both directly and indirectly to the patients. These activities have an affect on the ability of clinicians to provide quality care. Clinician-patient activities and other ancillary services crucial to the delivery of care to the patient such as radiology, pathology, and pharmacy services have a direct effect on patient's quality of care. Indirect influences of quality relate to the convenience, comfort, and safety of patients in the immediate environment of care. Administrative and technical services are also considered targets because they influence the performance of clinicians as they care for patients (e.g., informatics).

It is not just how the clinicians provide care for the patients that is scrutinized as a target for quality assurance, but also how the patients are able to provide care for themselves. Quality assurance even should include how the patient's family and friends will be involved in the healthcare delivery process. Knowing the complete process of healthcare delivery, including all the participants, enables failures to be detected in the delivery process and indicates where steps can be taken to improve patient care.

THE COMPONENTS OF QUALITY ASSURANCE

Donabedian divided quality assurance activities into two parts to explain functions and activities in healthcare delivery (Donabedian, 2003, XXV). The first part was called *system design and resources,* and the second part was called *performance monitoring and readjustment.* System design and resources included professional recruitment, education, training, and certification. It also included the number, distribution, equipment, organization, and licensure of hospitals and other healthcare facilities. Other areas of structure included the testing and marketing of drugs and biologicals, the financing of health care, access to healthcare goods and services, legal protection of consumer and provider interests, and so on.

Performance monitoring and readjustment is an activity by which one obtains information about the level of quality produced by the healthcare delivery system and, based on the interpretation of that information, takes the necessary actions to protect and improve quality health care to the patients. According to Donabedian (Donabedian, 2003, XXVII), the appropriate actions can take one of two forms. The first form educates and motivates people directly and the second form creates readjustments in system design and resources. The readjustments made are those that are expected to indirectly influence people's behavior. Anyone directly or indirectly involved in the delivery of health care can have their behavior influenced using this process methodology.

System design sets the average level of performance as well as the degree of variation above or below that average. By monitoring quality, the aim is to obtain a more precise adjustment of quality health care to the desired level. This is done by raising the average and reducing the variations around the new average. Quality monitoring is the activity by which the quality of healthcare delivery to the patients is being constantly observed. The saying goes, "one cannot manage what one doesn't measure." This is especially true in healthcare delivery.

THE QUALITY MONITORING CYCLE

Monitoring and readjustments are continuous activities. Donabedian described the quality monitoring cycle (Table 2-1) to include the following steps (Donabedian, 2003, XXVII): Obtaining data on performance; performing a pattern analysis—an epidemiological activity that identifies time, place, person, and function; providing an interpretation by advancing hypotheses that might explain the patterns observed; taking a preventive, corrective, or promotive action based on the causal hypotheses that have been advanced (i.e., resources, duties, functions, procedures, education); and obtaining data on subsequent performance to determine the consequences of the actions taken.

It is not the formality of providing a sequence of steps to quality monitoring but the message behind the process: observe, interpret, do something, assess what has been done, and repeat the cycle all over again and again. Quality monitoring is continuous just as healthcare delivery is an activity that never rests.

Quality monitoring is mainly a formal activity within a healthcare organization or a healthcare system. This formal, predictable monitoring activity is uniformly implemented and is acceptable to those whose practices it is meant to observe and scrutinize. Donabedian (Donabedian, 2003, XXIX)

Table 2-1   The Quality Monitoring Cycle

1. Obtain data on performance.
2. Perform pattern analysis—an epidemiological activity that identifies time, place, person, and function.
3. Provide interpretation by advancing hypotheses that might explain the patterns observed.
4. Take preventive, corrective, or promotive action based on the causal hypotheses that have been advanced (i.e., resources, duties, functions, procedures, education)
5. Obtain data on subsequent performance to determine the consequences of the actions taken.

Table created from material in Donabedian, A. *An introduction to quality assurance in health care*. New York, NY: Oxford University Press, Inc. 2003. pg. XXVII.

described a much more subtle, informal process that occurs when health-care clinicians observe each other at work and adjust their behavior to prevalent professional norms. The quality of health care can be greatly influenced by any activity that makes the work of clinicians visible to one another, to their students, and to all healthcare workers. These activities include collaborative work, referrals and consultations, clinical rounds, clinical pathology conferences, and other informal professional activities. It is these informal influences that may have the most impact on the delivery of health care to patients. Good practice will lead to copying of good practice by all and the reverse is also true, bad practice begets bad practice.

FOUNDATIONS OF QUALITY ASSURANCE

Donabedian described three foundations of quality assurance: commitment to quality, institutionalization of that commitment, and agreement on the meaning of quality (Donabedian, 2003, XXX). Commitment to quality requires a genuine commitment to process. The commitment cannot be simply a response to pressure from external sources (e.g., customers, community, etc.) to have a quality assurance program, but it must be internally motivated by pressures within the organization. A commitment must exist from everyone at all levels in the organization. Institutionalization of that commitment takes on a life of its own. Specific goals outline the organization's quality assurance program. An organizational structure for performance monitoring is created, and specifies both the chain of command and allocation of resources (people, time, place, money). Design and implementation of a set of formal monitoring activities are created and delineated to indicate what activities will be routine vs. occasional, centralized vs. decentralized. Mechanisms crucial to the short- and long-term success of the quality assurance program are created to communicate information and implement action. Most important in the institutionalization of the commitment to quality is creating a tradition or culture within the organization to strive for quality assurance. Everyone in the organization must acknowledge, accept, and practice quality assurance policies and procedures established all the time for the organization to be successful in this endeavor. The meaning or concept of quality in health care must and can be precisely defined, and is amenable to measurement; these measurements are accurate enough to be used as a basis for the effort to monitor and assure quality in healthcare delivery.

COMPONENTS OF QUALITY IN HEALTH CARE

Donabedian considered quality as the product of two factors (Donabedian, 2003, 4). One was the science and technology of health care. This included the biology of disease, behavioral attributes of the individual and population of patients, and diagnostic and therapeutic interventions. The second factor was the application of that science and technology in actual practice—the delivery of health care. The quality of care achieved in practice, according to Donabedian, was the product of these two factors. Donabedian went on to describe that product, quality in health care, by using several attributes (see Table 2-2) which included efficacy, effectiveness, efficiency, optimality, acceptability, legitimacy, and equity. These qualities, taken individually or in combination, constitute a definition of quality and, when measured in one way or another, will signify its magnitude.

Efficacy is the standard against which any improvement in health care achieved in actual practice is to be compared. Efficacy is not itself subject to monitoring when the quality of healthcare delivery is being assessed. Rather, according to Donabedian, "it is given to us, *a priori*," (Donabedian, 2003, 4) as a product of basic, clinical and applied medical research, experience, and professional consensus. An example of this is the randomized clinical control trial that will be discussed later in the book. The science and technology of health care set the standard for all the attributes of quality. This means that "actual performance in all aspects is compared to what our science and technology, at its best, is expected to achieve" (Donabedian, 2003, 4). The standards are not simply derived from science and technol-

---

Table 2-2   Donabedian's Seven Attributes of Quality in Health Care

1. Efficacy
2. Effectiveness
3. Efficiency
4. Optimality
5. Acceptability
6. Legitimacy
7. Equity

Table created from material in Donabedian, A. *An introduction to quality assurance in health care*. New York, NY: Oxford University Press, Inc. 2003. pg. 6.

ogy alone but they are also derived and set by social and individual preferences and some others by ethical and moral considerations.

Effectiveness is the degree to which attainable improvements in health and health care are attained (Donabedian, 2003, 7). It is a comparison between actual performance and the performance that the science and technology of health care, under most favorable or specified conditions, can be expected to achieve. In practical terms, the "relative effectiveness" is described as the improvements in health expected from the health care delivered to be assessed divided by the improvements in health to be expected from the "best" or "standard" of healthcare delivery established via evidence-based medicine.

A number of considerations help to clarify this attribute. Effectiveness is only relative to what the science and technology of health care can accomplish at any given time. Health care is limited by the changing landscape of new information, and as new discoveries in all aspects of healthcare delivery become established, the standard against which effectiveness is to be judged is raised accordingly.

The meaning and measure of effectiveness depends on how one defines and measures "health." Effectiveness is based on probabilities and not certainties. Individual cases or even a small number of cases in which a result has occurred cannot be properly measured. Rather, effectiveness is measured on what is expected to occur if an adequate sample of cases were to receive a specified kind of care. If a clinician gives care that is known to give the best results on the average in that kind of case, the care is judged to have been good enough regardless of patient outcome. Unfortunately, effectiveness is not fully appreciated because information about care is lacking, a poor definition of health is not agreed on, measures of health status are not agreed on, the course of untreated sickness is not known, the best or standard treatment is obscure, and documentation of outcomes is inadequate. This has become the motivation to perform more clinical trials and epidemiological studies in healthcare delivery to rectify these deficiencies.

Another way to improve on the measure of effectiveness is to apply it to whatever healthcare resources are available at the time of study. This in fact creates two scenarios—what is achievable with the best use of the resources at hand and what would be achievable with the best use of necessary resources.

Efficiency is the ability to lower the cost of care without diminishing attainable improvements in health (Donabedian, 2003, 9). It is defined as the expected improvements in health from the health care delivered to be assessed divided by the cost of that care. This means that efficiency in the delivery of health care is increased if, for a given cost of that care, health improvement is increased or if the same degree of health improvement is attained at a lower cost. Therefore, the reduction in cost does not denote efficiency unless health benefits are either unaffected or are improved.

There are three way of improving efficiency in health care. One way is to improve the *clinical efficiency* of healthcare deliverers. Increasing knowledge, judgment, and skill in the basic, clinical, and applied medical sciences leads to improvements in the actual delivery of health care. A second way to improve efficiency is to more efficiently produce the goods and/or services that are used in providing health care. This involves using the capital resources in healthcare delivery—space, equipment, and people—to provide care more efficiently. *Production or managerial efficiency* depends on organizational and managerial decisions in which clinicians do not play a decisive role (i.e., increasing the number of beds available for care in the hospital or using personnel to perform tasks that they are qualified to perform). The third way is provide health care more efficiently based on the sociodemographics of the patients being served (e.g., age, gender, ethnicity, economic status, and severity of illness) in a way proportionate to expected improvements in health. Resources are allocated to population subgroups that are perhaps sicker or are more likely to benefit from care, and do so for longer periods of time and at proportionately lower cost. This is called *distribution efficiency* and is an attribute of quality at the societal or population level.

Optimality is the balancing of improvements in health against the cost of such improvements (Donabedian, 2003, 11). There is a best or optimum relationship between costs and benefits of health care, a point below which more benefits could be obtained at costs that are low relative to the benefits, and above which additional benefits are obtained at costs too large relative to corresponding benefits. Clinicians are given successively larger sets of resources to use in healthcare delivery.

The issue is whether more is better. To a point, the more resources available, the more improved health care is delivered to patients. However, patients improvements begin to slow down despite the amount of resources available for their care. What happens at this point, called *optimally effective care,* is that the cost of care begins to outweigh the actual improvements to the patient; therefore resources are needlessly wasted and healthcare delivery in general does not benefit. *Maximally effective care* has been achieved when the clinician intuitively recognizes that no further improvement to the patient can be accomplished and requests no additional resources.

Donabedian believes in the importance of discussing cost with quality (Donabedian, 2003, 17), especially when clinicians provide health care more likely to be harmful than useful, or when health care provided is not necessarily harmful but useless. These types of healthcare delivery in the practice of medicine could be construed by the patient as being inattentive, careless, and ignorant of his/her personal needs. Donabedian further opines on this issue of cost and quality, "'useless' care for some leaves less for others who could have benefited from it, such care is socially irresponsible and therefore reprehensible" (Donabedian, 2003, 17).

Acceptability is defined as conformity to the wishes, desires, and expectations of patients and responsible members of their families (Donabedian, 2003, 18). This is also considered a "personal healthcare need" by the patient, and includes the patient's perception as to what is needed to remain healthy and free of illness, the cost to the patient to achieve total health and well-being, and whether the patient is willing to pay that cost. Donabedian explains this attribute in terms of the following main components: accessibility; the patient-clinician relationship; the amenities of care; patient preferences regarding the effects of health care received, the risks and costs of health care received; and what patients consider fair and equitable.

Accessibility deals with the ease with which a patient can obtain health care. This ease of access can depend on distances from the sources of care, availability of health care, and transportation to the source of care. The days and hours when sources of care are available to patients, the ability to pay for health care and/or insurability of the patients, and social and cultural factors also contribute to understanding accessibility of health care from both the individual and population perspective. Even the biases of those who are providing care can have an impact on accessibility. The patients and the community-at-large continue to be concerned about the ability to receive health care when it is desired and needed and with how easily and convenient the care can be obtained.

The clinician–patient relationship is critical to the acceptability of quality of health care. Personal concern, empathy, respectfulness, compassion, willingness to take time, informed consent for care, honesty, truthfulness, and attention to patient's preferences and "personal need" are all ingredients in providing high quality health care. Giving patients the inalienable right to choose their clinicians raises the bar for quality and enhances the healthcare delivery for patients and populations through clinician competition. Unfortunately, the 1980s and the advent of health maintenance organizations removed choice and competition from the marketplace, which only recently in the early 21st century is being returned to healthcare delivery in this country.

The amenities of care include properties such as convenience, privacy, comfort, restfulness, and cleanliness. This along with the clinician–patient relationship is what makes receiving health care either a pleasant and rewarding or unpleasant and humiliating experience. This aspect of care is not without some caveats. The amenities of care can be costly. Inefficiencies in the availability and delivery of technically and scientifically proven health care to patients and the community-at-large can also be masked. Often, the benefits derived from these added costs are based on comparison with alternative uses of the same resources and measuring the outcomes for the patients.

Patient's preferences regarding the consequences (effects, risks, and cost) of health care results in patient's regularly comparing the expected improvements in health to the risks associated with the healthcare delivered. Patients assign a value to each consequence of care. These are much different than the value their clinicians assign to each consequence. Patients' value of the consequences also differ significantly from each other. How can these differences be resolved?

Patient education, social financing, and ethical considerations can all help patients to decide whether a longer life with poor quality is preferred to a shorter life with higher quality. Informed decisions and patient-centered care are discussed in great detail as outcomes management is more fully explained later in the book.

The fair and equitable distribution of healthcare delivery is the final component to the discussion on acceptability. It is important to note that this is not the same as an equal distribution of healthcare delivery. An equal distribution of healthcare delivery means that everyone regardless of age, gender, and severity of illness would be expected to get the same amount of healthcare resources. Intuitively and morally, equality has long been recognized as having no place in the current healthcare delivery system for the previously discussed reasons.

Legitimacy is defined as conformity to social preferences, as expressed in ethical principles, values, norms, laws, and regulations (Donabedian, 2003, 22). Conformity to social preferences, also called social acceptability, is practiced in a democratic society that has a political system in place to represent the wishes, desires, and concerns of the people. Individual differences and differences between individuals and society as a whole in determining what kind of health care is most effective, efficient, optimal, and equitable can create a healthcare delivery system of indeterminate quality. Balancing individual's personal needs for health with the community-at-large is key for deciding how the healthcare delivery system can utilize.

Clinicians carry a heavy burden to execute the wishes of the legislated, regulated, and administrative decisions of a democratic society for public health and well-being (i.e., immunizations, sanitation, infectious disease control, etc.) with health consumerism, shared decision making, and patient-centered care. How does one decide for whom and at what time to use healthcare resources? Does the management of healthcare outcomes help to determine the answer to this question? Is individual or personal need any more important than the professional need of clinicians in determining how healthcare resources are to be used? Only a free society using social consensus can determine the answers to these and other questions of a similar context.

Equity is defined as conformity to a principle that determines what is just and fair in the distribution of healthcare delivery and of its benefits among the community-at-large (Donabedian, 2003, 24). Equity depends first on access to care, and second on the effectiveness and acceptability of the health care received. As a general rule, the differences between population groups should be minimized according to age, gender, income, education, ethnicity, and so on. Individual and social preferences should also be minimized. An equitable healthcare delivery system ensures certain categories of people have the care they need; these health improvements should be significant when compared to cost. The relative emphasis on preventive rather than therapeutic care is an example of this reasoning.

MONITORING AND IMPROVING CLINICAL PERFORMANCE

Assuring the quality of healthcare delivery by monitoring clinical performance and improving it when necessary was the major goal of Donabedian's life's work in healthcare management. He developed nine steps to follow to perform this endeavor (Donabedian, 2003, 27):

- Determining what to monitor
- Determining priorities in monitoring
- Selecting an approach (or approaches) to assessing performance

- Formulating criteria and standards
- Obtaining the necessary information
- Choosing when to monitor
- Choosing how to monitor
- Constructing a monitoring system
- Bringing about behavior change

Of these nine steps, selecting approaches to assessing performance is the most important to understanding healthcare outcomes management. There has to be some way of finding if the quality of care has been good, fair, or poor.

In the early 1970s, Donabedian (Donabedian, 2003, 46) describes three approaches to assessing the quality of care. Structure, process, and outcome: a triad that perhaps revolutionized the process of determining the quality of healthcare delivery for generations to come. Unfortunately, even though this model was simplistic, intuitive, and widely accepted, history reveals that it has not been well understood or even used properly.

STRUCTURE, PROCESS, AND OUTCOME

Structure designates the conditions under which health care is delivered. The conditions included may be *material resources,* such as facilities and equipment; *human resources and intellectual capital,* such as the number, variety, and qualifications of professional and support personnel; and

---

Table 2-3   The 9 Steps of Monitoring and Improving Clinical Performance

1. Determining what to monitor
2. Determining priorities in monitoring
3. Selecting an approach (or approaches) to assessing performance
4. Formulating criteria and standards
5. Obtaining the necessary information
6. Choosing when to monitor
7. Choosing how to monitor
8. Constructing a monitoring system
9. Bringing about behavior change

Table created from material in Donabedian, A. *An introduction to quality assurance in health care.* New York, NY: Oxford University Press, Inc. 2003. pg. 27.

organizational characteristics such as the medical and nursing staffs of a hospital or health system, management including supervision and performance review, and administrative functions including billing, accounts receivable, etc.

Process designates the activities that constitute the delivery of health care. This follows the continuum of care to include preventive care, acute care, chronic care, rehabilitative care, palliative care, and supportive care. The care is provided by clinicians and support personnel in a variety of settings including inpatient, outpatient, rehabilitative, and supportive centers of care.

Outcomes denote the changes in individuals and populations that can be attributed to healthcare delivery. Outcomes include changes in health status; in knowledge acquired by patients, family, and friends that may influence future delivery of health care; in behavior of patients, family, and friends that may influence future delivery of health care; in satisfaction of patients, family and friends with the health care received and its outcomes.

Donabedian (Donabedian, 2003, 47) is emphatic about the fact that structure, process, and outcome are not part of the "7" attributes of quality (see Table 2-2). They are only kinds of information obtained to help infer whether the studied quality of health care delivered was good or not. Inferences about the quality of health care delivered are not possible unless there is a predetermined relationship among the three approaches so that structure would influence process and process would then influence outcome.

There is not a clear beginning or ending in the relationship of the three approaches, nor is there a linear relationship that follows from structure to process to outcome. However, the ability to specify how a series of cause and effects is configured using the three approaches is much more important. This specification of analysis decides the data and information may be necessary to pass judgment on the quality of health care being delivered and how easily that information can be obtained.

Donabedian (Donabedian, 2003, 49) also indicates that the relations postulated to exist between adjacent pairs in the structure-process-outcome model are not certainties; rather they are probabilities. These probabilities may be large or small, and they may be well established by scientific evidence-based medicine or largely presumed. However, the higher the probabilities are and the more firmly established they are by scientific evidence-based medicine, the more credible the judgments about the quality of health care delivered can be. Donabedian (Donabedian, 2003, 49) further indicates that this model was established to assess clinical practice. The model may be used to evaluate other activities but its reliability and validity are questionable and up to the user to set parameters of study.

UNDERSTANDING HEALTHCARE OUTCOMES MANAGEMENT AND PLANNING USING DONABEDIAN'S MODEL

The best approach to understand the quality of healthcare delivery has been controversial for some time. According to Donabedian (Donabedian, 2003, 52), outcome assessment is favored over structure and process because it asserts that what matters most is the effect of the health care delivered on the patient's health and well-being. Donabedian cautions that if outcomes are used to make a judgment on the quality of the health care delivered, it should follow that the care being delivered and assessed is responsible for the outcome observed. Unfortunately, it is not always an easy correlation between cause and effect, antecedent health care delivered and subsequent outcomes. Donabedian has referred to this as the "problem of attribution" (Donabedian, 2003, 53).

The problem of attribution arises in part because the relationship between process and outcome is often not well understood and known. Even when the relationship between the two is known, the probability between cause and effect could be very small. The probabilistic nature between process and outcome means that in a small number of cases, there is no certainty that a given set of processes caused one or more of the outcomes to occur. Because this relationship is probabilistic, a larger number of cases are needed to establish a cause and effect relationship.

Even when a larger number of cases have been observed, there is further difficulty to overcome. Patients vary in their biological, psychological, social, and genetic characteristics. These are features well known to influence outcomes. Before some outcomes can stand on their own merit in assessing the quality of healthcare delivery, a correction must be made for these differences among patients. This is called "case-mix adjustment." There are many methods available to interpret case-mix adjustment (Thomas and Longo, 1990). However, Donabedian asserts (Donabedian,

2003, 53) that no complete methodology exists so that outcomes measurement can be relied on as the best approach for assessing the quality of health care delivered today.

Even though there may not be a perfect methodology, outcomes assessment gathers the contributions of all inputs of healthcare delivery from each source, including the contributions to the delivery of care by families and friends of the patients. Assigning to each input a weight proportionate to its contribution to the delivery of health care provides a distinct advantage over structure and process because these two approaches cannot easily do this. Outcomes assessment can also reflect how skillfully care was delivered to a patient. Many outcomes are subject to being felt and evaluated by patients, so they themselves can judge the quality of the care they receive.

Outcomes that occur during the course of healthcare delivery can be easily observed and assessed. It is by evaluating these observable outcomes that clinicians guide their conduct of healthcare delivery. An important issue arises when the outcome occurs after the care being delivered has terminated. The longer the time elapsed the more an opportunity exists for factors outside of health care to intervene, rendering the relationship between cause and effect, past healthcare delivery, and a remote outcome even more questionable.

The choice of how outcomes are to be measured determines whether the quality of health care delivered can be assessed appropriately. In this respect, Donabedian (Donabedian, 2003, 54) classifies outcomes as either "partial, diagnosis specific" or "inclusive, generic." Partial, specific outcomes are meant to tell us whether or not specific clinical objectives have been obtained in defined situations. For example, in a patient with high blood pressure, has a process been implemented to bring the patient's blood pressure into the normal range? Such measures are more dependent on the quality of health care delivered and more sensitive to variations in it. Inclusive, generic measures are meant to provide an estimate of health status without regard to diagnosis (Donabedian, 1973; Ware and Sherbourne, 1992). Mortality and longevity are two such measures. Longevity alone does not give a full picture of one's health and well-being. There are many well-accepted measures to assess patient functionality and quality of life available today (Leplege and Hunt, 1997; Wilson and Cleary, 1995) that provide degrees of longevity.

DONABEDIAN'S GUIDELINES FOR USING HEALTHCARE OUTCOMES MANAGEMENT AND PLANNING AS AN INDICATOR OF QUALITY HEALTHCARE DELIVERY

Donabedian provides important detailed guidelines as to how best to use outcome assessment as the preferred approach and indicator of quality healthcare delivery. First, the outcome selected should be relevant to the objective of health care being delivered. In other words, it should reflect what the clinician is aiming to accomplish. Second, the outcome must be achievable by "good" delivery of health care. The methods for providing this good healthcare delivery must be available and under the control of the clinicians providing services in the healthcare delivery system. Third, the outcome, whether "good" or "bad," must be attributable first to the health care being delivered, and then to the contribution of the clinician whose performance is being assessed. Fourth, the duration of the outcome as well as its magnitude should be taken into account. Fifth, the trade-off between levels and durations of alternative outcomes may be considered. A shorter life at a higher level of function may have to be weighed against a longer life with greater impairment and disability. Sixth, the information on the relevant outcome must be available. This is not always easy, especially when the necessary information on the outcome must be obtained over extended periods of time. Seventh, the consequences of taking action and also the consequences of not taking action must be tracked to obtain a complete picture of performance. Finally, the outcome cannot stand alone. The means used to achieve the outcome must be considered unless it is assumed that healthcare resources are unlimited, which is often untrue.

DONABEDIAN'S CLASSIFICATIONS OF OUTCOMES

Donabedian provides a complete classification of outcomes (see Table 2-4) in keeping with his three approaches to assessing quality in healthcare delivery (Donabedian, 1982). He describes seven categories for consideration that go beyond the three broader categories previously discussed. The categories are: clinical, physiological-biochemical, physical, psychological-mental, social and psychological, integrative outcomes, and evaluative outcomes.

Table 2-4   Donabedian's Classifications of Outcomes

---

1. Clinical
2. Physiological-biochemical
3. Physical
4. Psychological-mental
5. Social and psychological
6. Integrative
7. Evaluative

Table created from material in Donabedian, A. *An introduction to quality assurance in health care.* New York, NY: Oxford University Press, Inc. 2003. pg. 48.

The *clinical* classification of outcomes includes patient-reported symptoms that have clinical significance—diagnostic categorization as an indication of morbidity, disease staging relevant to functional changes and prognosis and diagnostic performance or the frequency of false positives and false negatives as indicators of good, fair, or poor results.

The *physiological-biochemical* classification includes the abnormalities defined and reported through diagnostic and ancillary testing. This describes loss of biological functionality and impairment in the body's functional reserve in test situations under various degrees of stress.

The *physical* classification of outcomes includes the loss or impairment of structural form or integrity and includes anatomical abnormalities, defects, and disfigurements. This also includes changes in functional performance of physical activities and tasks under the activities of daily living and under test conditions that involve various degrees of stress to the body.

The *psychological-mental* classification of outcomes describes patient's feelings of discomfort, pain, fear, and anxiety or their opposites. Patient beliefs that are relevant to health care or individual personal needs, knowledge that is relevant to healthful living, healthcare delivery, and coping mechanisms during illness are also included in this outcome. Impairments of discrete psychological or mental functionality under the activities of daily living and under test conditions that involve various degrees of stress to the body are also included in this category.

The *social and psychological* classification of outcomes includes patient's behaviors that are relevant to coping with current illness or affect future health status, including adherence to healthcare regimens and changes in health-related habits. This category identifies different roles that patients play during illness and includes them in the analysis of outcomes (e.g., spousal, familial, occupational, and interpersonal).

The *integrative outcomes* have been discussed briefly already and include mortality and longevity with adjustments made to take into account impairments of physical, psychological, or psychosocial function. The monetary value of mortality and longevity are also accounted for in this outcome category.

The *evaluative outcomes* are subjective opinions from patients, family, and friends about satisfaction with various aspects of healthcare delivery including accessibility, continuity, thoroughness, humaneness, informativeness, effectiveness, and cost.

Although Donabedian attempts to bring a complete classification to healthcare outcomes, this classification scheme is open to interpretation and to other contextual beliefs and values from the clinician, patient, family, and friends' perspective. It is important to frame the reference of discussion when using these categories to discuss healthcare outcomes management as the perspective in which the discussion ensues can radically change what is included as an endpoint when quality in healthcare delivery is assessed.

Healthcare Delivery in the 21st Century— A Report from the Institute of Medicine

INTRODUCTION TO THE REPORT

The Institute of Medicine has defined quality as "the degree to which health services for individuals and populations increase the likelihood of desired health outcomes and are consistent with current professional knowledge" (Lohr, 1990). Good quality means providing patients with appropriate services in a technically competent manner, with good communication, shared decision making, and cultural sensitivity (Institute of Medicine, 2001). These definitions originated when the Committee on the Quality of Health Care in America was formed in June, 1998. This committee was charged with developing a strategy that would substantially improve the quality of healthcare delivery in the United States over the next 10 years. (Institute of Medicine, 2001, 1) What led to the development of this committee? Had not the lessons of quality improvement that developed in Japan, or the 30 years of work led by Donabedian in dissecting quality assurance in healthcare delivery in the United States, gone totally ignored? Would we ever begin to understand healthcare outcomes management in a way that resulted in value to patients, families, and friends? How would healthcare delivery in the United States begin to harm patients less frequently and routinely deliver great benefits to the stakeholders? It was clearly recognized prior to forming the committee that a great chasm had developed between the health care available to Americans at the end of the 20th century and the health care that could be delivered in the 21st century.

The committee, in carrying out its charge for developing a strategy for quality improvement in healthcare delivery, performed the following tasks (Institute of Medicine, 2000, 1-2):

1. Commissioned a detailed review of the literature on the quality of care
2. Convened a communications workshop to identify strategies for raising awareness of the general public and key stakeholders of quality concerns
3. Identified environmental forces that encourage or impede efforts to improve quality
4. Developed strategies for fostering greater accountability for quality
5. Identified important areas of research that should be pursued to facilitate improvements in quality

The committee focused on the personal (individual) healthcare delivery system, specifically, the provision of preventive, acute, chronic, and end-of-life health care. Population health was not a major focus for the committee in fulfilling its mission. Population medicine and its role in the delivery of quality and healthcare outcomes management is addressed later in the book.

The committee published their first report, *To Err is Human: Building a Safer Health System* (Institute of Medicine, 2000), as an effort to address patient safety. The committee concluded that tens of thousands of Americans die needlessly each year from harmful errors in healthcare delivery and that hundreds of thousands suffer or barely escape from nonfatal injuries that a high quality healthcare delivery system would largely prevent.

Safety was only one of the major issues of quality in healthcare delivery addressed by the committee. Other issues of quality in healthcare delivery addressed by the committee included health, functioning, dignity, comfort, satisfaction, and resources of Americans. This second report on the state of quality healthcare delivered in the United States is a call for action to improve the American healthcare delivery system as a whole, in all its quality dimensions, for all Americans (Institute of Medicine, 2001).

THE NEED FOR CHANGE

Research on the quality of healthcare delivery reveals that the American health care system cannot adequately translate new medical knowledge into clinical practice and cannot apply new technology safely and appropriately. A review of the literature commissioned by the National Coalition on Health Care in 1997 (Schuster, McGlynn, and Brook, 1998) revealed more than 70 publications in peer-reviewed journals have documented serious quality shortcomings. Variations in performance across the healthcare delivery system were identified in various patient care venues. The delivery of health care has become fragmented and no strong clinical informatics exist to collect, store, and interpret healthcare data. Consequently, poorly designed healthcare processes exist, characterized by inefficient use of resources and inadequate access to healthcare delivery. Most importantly, the literature points to significant risks of harm to patients and poorer patient outcomes (Chassin and Gavin, 1998; Schuster et al., 1998).

The last part of the 20th century recognized mergers, acquisitions, and affiliations as the main focus for healthcare delivery in the United States. As changes in the mechanisms of payment for healthcare services evolved, contraction of the healthcare delivery system occurred, yet little was done to actually change the delivery process.

More and more Americans are faced with increasing responsibility for their health care (e.g., payment for services received) and employers are decreasing their contribution to employees' healthcare benefits. Leaders of healthcare delivery are being challenged to plan for the future while simultaneously trying to deal with reductions in third party payments, inadequate nurse staffing, and growing uninsured Americans seeking uncompensated healthcare delivery (Institute of Medicine, 2000).

Chronic medical conditions have become the leading causes of illness, disability, and death in this country today. Half of the United States population is affected by chronic, preventable disease and accounts for the majority of healthcare expenditures (Hoffman et al., 1996). More than 40 percent of patients with chronic disease have more than one chronic disease for which they are being treated (The Robert Wood Johnson Foundation, 1996).

Unfortunately for patients, clinicians often work independently of one another and patient information is not shared in a timely fashion to have a positive impact on the outcomes of clinical care (e.g., medical history, services provided in various venues, pharmaceuticals given to patients, etc.).

The need for change in America's healthcare delivery system is greater now than ever before. The fact that issues related to patient safety and poor clinical outcomes are being uncovered require the country to respond expeditiously. However, the fix doe not lie with the people working in the healthcare delivery system. The answer to solving the many problems of healthcare delivery today is truly in the process of delivery of the care. As Shewhart, Deming, Juran, and Donabedian have indicated, the problem with achieving high quality and good outcomes falls within the confines of the system; rarely are people the reason for poor results. The need for leadership and direction in health care is of the utmost importance.

The committee on the Quality of Health Care in America (Institute of Medicine, 2001) proposed an agenda for redesigning the 21st century healthcare system:

- All health constituencies (Table 1-1) must commit to a national statement of purpose for the healthcare system as a whole and to a shared agenda of six aims for improvement that can raise the quality of care to unprecedented levels.
- All health constituencies that support healthcare delivery must adopt a new set of principles to guide the redesign of healthcare processes.
- The government agencies responsible for the healthcare delivery system in the United States must identify a set of priority conditions upon which to focus initial efforts, provide resources to stimulate innovation, and initiate the change process.
- Organizations in the healthcare delivery system must design and implement more effective organizational support processes to make change in the delivery of health care possible.
- All health constituencies must create an environment that fosters and rewards improvement by:
  - Creating an infrastructure to support evidence-based medicine.
  - Facilitating the use of information technology.
  - Aligning payment incentives.
  - Preparing the workforce to better serve patients in a world of expanding knowledge and rapid change (Institute of Medicine, 2001).

ESTABLISHING AIMS FOR THE 21ST CENTURY HEALTHCARE DELIVERY SYSTEM

The committee on Quality of Health Care in America (Institute of Medicine, 2001) proposed six aims for improvement (see Table 3-1) to address key dimensions in which today's healthcare delivery system functions at far lower levels than it should. The committee proposed that healthcare delivery should be:

- *Safe* by avoiding injuries to patients from the delivered health care intended to help them.
- *Effective* by providing healthcare services based on scientific knowledge to all who could benefit and by refraining from providing services to those not likely to benefit (avoiding underuse and overuse, respectively).
- *Patient-centered* by providing care that is respectful of and responsive to individual patient preferences, needs, and values and ensuring that patient values guide all clinical decisions.
- *Timely* by reducing waiting periods and sometimes harmful delays for both those who receive healthcare services and those who provide those services.
- *Efficient* by avoiding waste in the valuable resources available to all health constituents (i.e., equipment, supplies, ideas, intellectual capital, and energy).
- *Equitable* by providing care that does not vary in quality because of personal characteristics such as gender, ethnicity, geography, and socioeconomic status (Institute of Medicine, 2001).

Table 3-1   Six Aims for Improvement in Healthcare Delivery

1. Safe
2. Effective
3. Patient-centered
4. Timely
5. Efficient
6. Equitable

Table created from material in Institute of Medicine. Crossing the Quality Chasm: A New Health System for the 21st Century. Washington, D.C.: National Academy Press, 2001. pg. 5–6.

A healthcare delivery system that could achieve major gains in the six dimensions would be far more successful in meeting patient's needs and improving healthcare outcomes. The committee believed that patients, their families, and friends would realize safer healthcare delivery that would be more reliable, responsive, more integrated, and more available. The continuum of care would be made available to all patients regardless of their entry point into the healthcare delivery system (e.g., acute, chronic, preventive, rehabilitative, or end-of-life care). Clinicians would be able to provide more coordinated, integrated health care with an emphasis on sharing information and having the technology to provide safer, more reliable and responsive healthcare services.

Progress in achieving these six aims must be well tracked so healthcare delivery can continue to improve. Knowing the beginning, the middle, and the end of the process is crucial so successes in reaching high quality healthcare delivery can be shared with the American public. All health constituencies must believe that the changes being made are actually making a difference, and result in safer care and improved healthcare outcomes. The committee is quick to note that even though their report focused healthcare delivery for the individual patient, the six aims for improvement are sufficiently robust that they can be applied equally to decisions and evaluations at the population health level (Institute of Medicine, 2001).

FORMULATING NEW RULES TO REDESIGN AND IMPROVE CARE

Innovation in health care lies at the heart of redesigning and improving healthcare delivery. Empowering patients, families, friends, and clinicians to step out of their comfort zones and to communicate new ideas to improve quality and outcomes is key to this redesign. Much of the redesign must be done incrementally and it must occur at the local level of healthcare delivery. National and state levels of legislation, regulation, and administration have demonstrated over the past 60 years that the healthcare bureaucracy is incapable of innovation. Redesign must be done by looking at the processes within the system. Utilizing the intellectual capital within each small delivery system is a critical success factor for redesigning and improving healthcare delivery.

The committee on Quality of Health Care in America (Institute of Medicine, 2001) has been guided by the belief that high quality health care must be delivered by carefully and consciously designed healthcare delivery systems that provide healthcare services that are *safe, effective, patient-centered, timely, efficient,* and *equitable.* Such systems, according to the committee, must be designed to serve the needs of patients, and to ensure that they are fully informed, retain control, and participate in healthcare delivery whenever possible, and that patients receive health care that is respectful of their values and preferences. Such delivery systems must apply evidence-based medicine to clinical practice and allow clinicians to attain the tools and supports to deliver consistent, safe healthcare services.

The committee encourages all healthcare constituencies to redesign healthcare processes in accordance with the following rules:

1. *Care based on continuous healing relationships.* Patients should receive health care whenever and wherever it is needed. The healthcare system needs to be responsive and ensure access 24 hours per day, 365 days per year (e.g., face-to-face, telephonic, and over the Internet).

2. *Customization based on patient needs and values.* Individual patient choices and preferences should be addressed along with the healthcare delivery system preparing to meet the most common basic needs of most patients.

3. *The patient as the source of control.* Patients should be given the necessary information and the opportunity to exercise the degree of control they choose over healthcare decisions that affect them. The healthcare delivery system should be able to accommodate differences in patient preferences and encourage shared decision making.

4. *Shared knowledge and the free flow of information.* Patients should have easy access to their own personal medical information as well as have access to clinical knowledge. Patients, family, friends, and clinicians should share information and communicate effectively and efficiently.

5. *Evidence-based decision making.* Patients should receive healthcare services that are based on valid and reliable clinical results with minimal variability from clinician-to-clinician.

6. *Safety as a system priority.* Patients should be safe from injury and illness caused by the healthcare delivery system itself. Reducing risk

and ensuring patient safety require greater attention to systems that help prevent and mitigate errors in healthcare service delivery.

7. *The need for transparency.* Patients, family, and friends should be given information by healthcare delivery systems and clinicians to allow for informed decision making when selecting a health plan, healthcare system, provider, and treatment, including all alternative treatments. Information about safety, evidence-based medicine, and patient satisfaction should be made available at all times when requested.

8. *Anticipation of needs.* The importance of being proactive along with being reactive is necessary for meeting patient needs and preferences.

9. *Continuous decrease in waste.* The healthcare delivery system should not waste any of its resources used in supplying services to patients, family, and friends (e.g., land, labor, equipment, and intellectual capital).

10. *Cooperation among clinicians.* Clinicians and the institutions within which they work should have an "esprit de corps" that fosters collegiality, scholarship, communication, collaboration, coordination, and compassion (Institute of Medicine, 2001).

These ten rules should lead the healthcare delivery system in the direction of redesign and improvement. Promoting innovation and the redesign of healthcare delivery is required to achieve the aims of improvement outlined by the committee. These rules are grounded in both logic and varying degrees of evidence, and according to the committee, will represent a new paradigm for healthcare delivery. These rules must be constantly reassessed and realigned so progress toward meeting the aims of improvement and the special effects attributable to the ten rules themselves can be successful. These rules should be adopted where possible so that the change of culture needed by the healthcare delivery system can occur and can impact patient safety and outcomes of healthcare delivered.

IMPROVING OUTCOMES OF COMMON CONDITIONS

Applying the ten rules for process redesign of the current healthcare delivery system in the United States is only the beginning of the many necessary changes required to improve the outcomes of health care. The committee on Quality of Health Care in America (Institute of Medicine,

2001) recognizes the requirement of a widespread application of process redesign and a commitment to evidence-based medicine that is responsive to individual patient's needs and preferences. Well-designed and fully implemented healthcare delivery systems are required to achieve positive outcomes. For this to occur public policy and private market forces must align. The appropriate information technology infrastructure must support this process change to ensure successful implementation. The committee notes that to initiate the process changes necessary for success, the healthcare delivery system must focus more on the development of healthcare processes for the common conditions that afflict Americans today. Only fifteen to twenty five chronic conditions account for the majority of healthcare services delivered today (Ray, 2000). The majority of the common conditions are chronic disease states.

Health care for chronic diseases is much different than the care for acute and self-limited medical conditions. Care for the chronically ill needs to be multidimensional and collaborative. Effective communication among clinicians and between clinicians and patients, their families, and friends, is critical to providing high quality health care for patients with chronic disease. Personal health information must accompany patients as they transition among all healthcare venues in which they receive care (e.g., home, office, hospital, etc.).

Meticulously designed, evidence-based care processes supported by automated clinical information and decision-support systems, offer the greatest potential for achieving the best outcomes from care for chronic conditions. Evidence-based medicine has been creating clinical pathways and guidelines for standardized care for some time (Eisenberg, 2000). Unfortunately, even though evidence-based medicine is available for all clinicians today, the quality of care and the outcomes from the health care received by the patient remains with considerable variability for many chronic diseases. The committee feels strongly that with the current variations in both healthcare quality and outcomes, and the prevalence of chronic conditions, chronic diseases represent an excellent starting point for efforts to better define optimum healthcare delivery and to design healthcare delivery processes to meet current patient needs and preferences.

The committee noted that all the health constituencies in today's healthcare delivery system should work together to organize evidence-based medicine consistent with best practices, organize major preventive healthcare programs to target key health-risk behaviors associated with the onset or progression of the chronic diseases, design and develop an information infrastructure to support the provision of healthcare services and the ongoing measurement of healthcare processes and patient outcomes, and align the incentives inherent in the current payment schemes and accountability processes with the goal of quality improvement.

The redesign and implementation of well-designed healthcare processes for priority chronic conditions requires a great deal of resources. Land, labor, equipment, and intellectual capital are required to enhance organizational capacity, to build an information infrastructure, and to train multidisciplinary healthcare delivery teams. Private and public funding institutions must step up for this to take place. Initially, funding should be directed to the programs that will have early successes. However, as time passes, efforts to improve the quality of care and patient outcomes must be directed to the conditions that require more resources to reach success. The public sector cannot handle the burden of being the primary benefactor for the redesign of healthcare delivery processes. The private sector must shoulder the majority of the costs for resources because of the financial peril that the public sector continues to experience today and into the future.

ORGANIZATIONAL SUPPORTS FOR CHANGE

A healthcare delivery system that is responsive to patients' needs and preferences and uses evidence-based medicine requires an organization that is flexible and innovative. Hospitals, physician practices, integrated delivery systems, and health plans today remain unable to demonstrate a commitment to innovation and flexibility for patient healthcare delivery. The committee on Quality of Health Care in America (Institute of Medicine, 2001) identifies five major challenges for healthcare organizations that support change in healthcare delivery for the 21st century:

- Redesign of healthcare processes based on evidence-based medicine to serve more effectively and efficiently the needs of the chronically ill in a seamless, coordinated effort across healthcare settings and clinicians over time.
- Use of information technologies to improve access to clinical information and support clinical decision making for the patient, family, friends, and all healthcare constituencies.

- Manage the growing knowledge base and ensure that all those in the healthcare workforce have the skills and training required to maintain licensure, accreditation, and competency.
- Coordinate the delivery of healthcare services to patients across the continuum of care over time in a seamless manner.
- Incorporate performance and outcome measurements for improvement and accountability of the healthcare delivery system (Institute of Medicine, 2001).

ESTABLISHING A NEW ENVIRONMENT FOR HEALTHCARE DELIVERY

The committee on Quality of Health Care in America (Institute of Medicine, 2001) notes that to enable the profound changes in healthcare delivery recommended in their report, the environment of care must also change. The committee identified two types of environmental change. The first change focuses and aligns the environment toward the six aims for improvement (see Table 3-1). Payers must eliminate or modify payment practices that fragment the healthcare delivery system. Incentives should be established to encourage and reward innovation in healthcare delivery services aimed at improving quality. The creation of precise streams of accountability and measurement reflecting achievements in the six aims must be required by purchasers and regulators. Most importantly, healthcare consumers need to be guided in understanding the six aims, why they are important to healthcare delivery, and how to interpret the levels of performance of various healthcare delivery systems. The second change provides, where possible, assets and encouragement for positive change. Formal programs exchanging best practices need to be adopted both nationally and regionally. Research on new designs for the care of chronic conditions needs to be funded. A national system for monitoring the progress toward the six aims for improvement must also be established.

The committee recommends the above environmental changes need to occur in the following four major areas: the infrastructure that supports the dissemination and application of new clinical knowledge and technologies; the information technology infrastructure; payment policies; and the preparation of the healthcare delivery workforce. Changes in the quality oversight and accountability processes of public and private purchasers of healthcare services are also necessary.

APPLYING EVIDENCE TO HEALTHCARE DELIVERY

The committee (Institute of Medicine, 2001) recognizes that in the current healthcare delivery system, scientific knowledge about best practice is not applied systematically or expeditiously to clinical medical practice. An average of 17 years is required for new knowledge generated by randomized controlled trials to be incorporated into clinical medical practice, and even then application of best practice is highly uneven (Balas and Boren, 2000). Variability in clinical medical practice in which there is strong scientific evidence and a high degree of expert consensus about best practices indicates that current dissemination efforts fail to reach many clinicians and patients. There are insufficient tools and incentives to promote rapid adoption of best practices.

A more effective infrastructure where knowledge and technology can be applied must be designed, developed, implemented, and adopted by all healthcare delivery systems for the environment of care to change. In addition, the committee believes that the leadership of all the constituencies involved in healthcare delivery should focus initially on priority conditions and include ongoing analysis and synthesis of the medical evidence, delineation of specific clinical practice guidelines, identification of best practices in the design of healthcare delivery processes, enhanced dissemination efforts to communicate evidence and guidelines to the general public and professional communities, development of decision support tools to assist clinicians and patients in applying the evidence-based medicine, and the development of quality measures for priority chronic medical conditions.

USING INFORMATION TECHNOLOGY

The revolution of medical informatics and healthcare information technology management has had little impact on the healthcare delivery system to date. The therapeutic relationship between a clinician and patient is a relationship based on the exchange of clinical information; the patient shares information with the clinician about his/her general health, symptoms, and concerns and clinicians use their knowledge and skill sets to respond with both pertinent clinical medical information and reassurance.

The medical record is the current way clinical medical information about the life and times of the patient is stored. Poorly organized and often illegible, the medical record is rarely updated on a real-time basis to reflect real-time changes that have occurred in the patients care within the healthcare delivery system. This creates a barrier between the clinician and the patient that potentially results in poor quality outcomes and significant cost inefficiencies.

The design, development, and application of more sophisticated clinical information systems is essential to enhance the quality of care received by patients and to improve efficiencies within the healthcare delivery system. The Internet has enormous potential to transform the delivery of healthcare services through clinical information technology applications in such areas as consumer health, clinical care, administrative and financial transactions, population and public health, professional education, and biomedical and health services research (National Research Council, 2000).

The committee (Institute of Medicine, 2001) believes clinical information technology must play a central role in the redesign of healthcare delivery systems if a substantial improvement in quality is to be achieved in the next decade. Automation of clinical, administrative, and financial transactions is essential to improving quality, preventing errors, enhancing consumer confidence in the healthcare delivery system, and improving efficiency. The secure transfer of electronic information is already being instituted in many of venues of healthcare delivery. The Health Insurance Portability and Accountability Act (HIPAA) of 1996 is well underway in requiring all healthcare constituencies to follow legislated, regulated, and administrative guidelines that protect the patient's information in all clinical, administrative, and financial transactions. Unfortunately, adoption of clinical information technology is hampered by the skepticism and ignorance of the clinicians who prefer the antiquated paper system of today's healthcare delivery system.

Patient adoption and clinician acceptance require leadership from all the healthcare constituencies if clinical information technology is to move forward in the next decade. Again, the goal is to improve the quality of healthcare services delivered to patients and to improve on efficiencies in the care processes.

ALIGNING PAYMENT POLICIES WITH QUALITY IMPROVEMENT

Current payment practices do not adequately encourage or support the provision of high quality healthcare services today. Although payment practices are not the only factor that influences clinician and patient behavior, it remains an important piece of establishing a new environment for care.

All payment methodologies affect behavior and quality. Fee-for-service payment methodologies potentially encourage the *overuse* of healthcare services on the part of clinicians. These are healthcare services that may not be necessary within the standard of care or may expose the patient to more harm than good. Capitation and case payment methodologies potentially encourage the *underuse* of healthcare services. These are healthcare services that are not provided to patients, but may have great benefit to the patient's health and well being. There are no payment practices that will perfectly align financial incentives with the goal of providing high quality, cost effective healthcare services for all the health constituencies.

The committee (Institute of Medicine, 2001) believes that all health constituencies should examine the current payment practices and remove barriers that impede quality improvement to build stronger incentives for quality enhancement. Payment methodologies should provide fair payment for good clinical management of the types of patients seen. Fair practice should compensate clinicians for all types of patients, regardless of age, gender, or severity of disease. In addition, payment methodologies should provide an opportunity for clinicians to share in the benefits of quality improvement. Rewards should be located close to the level at which the reengineering and process redesign improved the quality of healthcare services delivered. These payment methodologies should also provide the opportunity for consumers and purchasers of healthcare services to recognize differences in healthcare delivery and direct their decisions accordingly. Education and training in quality are necessary for these constituencies to assist them to use their new-found knowledge and skill set in making good, informed choices for their patients' care. Financial incentives should be aligned with the implementation of healthcare processes based on evidence-based medicine, best practices, and the achievement of better patient outcomes. Clinicians need incentives to be motivated and should be rewarded for carefully designing, developing, and implementing healthcare processes that achieve higher levels of safety, effectiveness, patient-centeredness, timeliness, efficiency, and equity. Finally, these payment methodologies should reduce the fragmentation of healthcare services. Payment practices should not serve as a barrier to clinicians' ability to coordinate the healthcare services of their patients across the venues of healthcare delivery and over time.

The committee believes that in order to achieve a change in the current payment practices, opportunities exist through innovation in applying new payment methodologies. This includes blended methods of payment for clinicians (i.e., fee-for-service vs. capitation vs. case rates), multiyear contracts, payment modifications to encourage use of electronic methods among clinicians and between clinicians and patients, risk adjustment, bundled payments for priority conditions, and alternative approaches for addressing the capital investments needed to improve quality and process in healthcare delivery.

PREPARING THE WORKFORCE

To move into the 21st century of healthcare delivery, the committee believes that the healthcare workforce needs to develop new skills and knowledge in ways of relating to patients, their families, and friends, as well as to each other. The committee recommends three approaches be taken to accomplish this task. First, redesign the way health professionals are trained throughout the continuum of training (i.e., undergraduate, graduate, and continuing medical education) to emphasize the aims for improvement discussed earlier in this chapter. This would include teaching evidence-based medicine, population medicine, and best practices using a multidisciplinary approach. Second, modify the ways in which health professionals are regulated to facilitate the changes needed in healthcare delivery. State medical boards need to reevaluate and modify regulations to allow for innovation in the use of all types of clinicians so patients needs can be met in the most effective and efficient manner possible. Credentialing and certification procedures need to adopt new methods to keep up with the modifications required to provide high quality, cost effective healthcare services. Third, examine how the medical liability system can constructively support changes in healthcare delivery while remaining part of an overall approach to accountability for clinicians and healthcare organizations.

SUMMARY

The healthcare delivery system and all the health constituencies involved in healthcare delivery must realize the need for sweeping changes to improve the quality of care and outcomes for patients. The committee on Quality of Health Care in America (Institute of Medicine, 2001) envisions the 21st century healthcare system to be evidence-based, patient-centered, and systems/process oriented. New roles and responsibilities will exist for clinicians and patients, their families, and friends. A consumer-driven healthcare model that requires shared decision making will be necessary, along with innovation for education of clinicians at all levels of training in evidence-based and population medicine that is patient-centered, cost effective, and electronically mediated.

Systems Approach to Healthcare Outcomes Management

INTRODUCTION TO SYSTEMS IN HEALTH CARE

Beginning immediately after World War II, America faced three major revolutions in healthcare delivery. First, private employer-sponsored health insurance was introduced in the late 1940s to keep American workers from leaving their jobs and moving to the competition. Second, the United States government in the early 1960s introduced Medicare and Medicaid to assist America's elderly and disabled in obtaining the necessary healthcare services to survive. Finally, the early 1980s brought about an innovative approach to healthcare delivery known to all as "managed care." Each one of these major revolutions initiated profound changes in healthcare delivery that has led American employers, payers, and consumers to an unknown future for the delivery of healthcare services in the United States today.

As Americans enter the 21st century, an evolution in healthcare delivery is slowly developing. There are no major government healthcare services programs waiting to be unveiled to the public. The one-time administrative efficiencies and cost savings brought to American employers via managed care in the early 1990s have been used by over 90 percent of U.S. corporations and companies to date. Consumers have educated themselves in healthcare delivery and have begun to exercise their options by demanding better customer service that focuses on quality, cost, and accessibility. The time has come for the suppliers of healthcare services to embrace change and to accept the challenges that await us all in the 21st century.

Innovative medical technology and services have changed both the amount of health care available to patients today, and how it is delivered. Exponential growth of healthcare facilities and practitioners has changed the venue for the delivery of healthcare services from a traditional hospital setting to a variety of outpatient settings. Unfortunately, the planning and evaluation of medical technology and treatment remains controversial today. Because neither patients nor clinicians fully understand healthcare outcomes management, a number of different approaches exist to satisfy both the health consumer's and professional's need for knowledge.

Historically, planning and evaluation of outcomes has relied on the intuition and subjective assessment of clinicians. Personal experience and clinical anecdotes were shared behind closed doors (e.g., at the Morbidity and Mortality Conference) amongst physicians only to further the progress of medical treatment and to apply peer pressure to conform to acceptable standards of care for the times. However, the patient, family, and friends were never allowed to directly participate in these closed sessions of discovery and learn about the practice of medicine from the professional's point of view. In fact, it had long been accepted medical practice for the patient, their family, and friends, to blindly navigate through the healthcare delivery system guided only by the trust and faith in their clinician to do no harm.

A number of factors have changed the way healthcare outcomes management has been studied and taught. A shift toward a more scientific approach to the planning and evaluation of healthcare outcomes has evolved in the past few years as a result of the growth in medical errors. These errors have resulted in serious harm to patients, unsuccessful medical procedures that have resulted in an increase in morbidity and mortality, and an awareness that healthcare resources (e.g., land, labor, equipment, and intellectual capital) are very limited and that demand for these services in the American healthcare delivery system are unlimited. The cost of healthcare delivery has taken center stage along with patient satisfaction and quality of life issues.

Cochrane (Cochrane, 1972) argued that the: "Development of effective and efficient health services needs hard evidence, preferably based upon randomized trials, that the application of each procedure either alters the natural history of disease in appreciable proportion of patients or otherwise benefits them at reasonable cost." Additionally, healthcare delivery has functioned without a modern information infrastructure that rigorously and efficiently connects all those who generate, store, distribute, transfer, and use medical information to those who need the proper application of that information and knowledge. At the crux of the problem in healthcare outcomes management is the need to develop a process that systematically defines and describes the four major areas of concern:

- Clinical performance
- Financial performance
- Individual and population-health functionality and quality of life
- Patient satisfaction with healthcare delivery received

This requires a more complete understanding of how subjective and objective data collection can occur simultaneously and in harmony for outcomes information to have meaning and purpose.

Unfortunately, the drivers of healthcare inflation (see Table 4-1) have caused the process to be delayed for almost three decades. These drivers have shifted the healthcare delivery system into a crisis mode that has resulted in a change in focus to rebuilding profits and less on building market share for services to be supplied to patients. In fact, the development of a "kinder and gentler" healthcare delivery system has given way to a more corporate mentality: "No margin, no mission." The actual reality in America's healthcare delivery system today is: "No measure, no margin." However, what many healthcare delivery systems have realized is that the drivers of healthcare inflation caused in a shift in the burden of paying for healthcare services back to the patient. Thus, a movement of consumerism and a demand by patients to have more control over their healthcare activities has emerged.

Table 4-1   Drivers of Healthcare Inflation

1. General price inflation
2. Biotechnology advances
    i. Cost
3. Consumer demand
    i. Over-utilization of healthcare resources
    ii. Choice
    iii. Lack of responsible personal health status
    iv. Unrealistic expectations of the healthcare system
4. Pharmaceutical costs
    i. Research & development
    ii. Marketing
    iii. Branding
5. Demographic changes
    i. Aging population
    ii. Uninsured/underinsured
6. Cost shifting
    i. Public to private
        1. Below cost government program reimbursement
    ii. Patient "Bill of Rights"
7. New health insurance underwriting cycle
    i. Hard phase
        1. Rebuilding profits
        2. Decrease emphasis on market share
    ii. Lack of substantial insurer competition
        1. Soft phase
8. Malpractice claims
    i. Litigation costs
    ii. Defensive medicine
9. Lifestyle disease
10. Cost of care
    i. Poor quality
    ii. Inappropriate care
    iii. Dramatically different practice patterns utilized by providers
    iv. Over supply of facilities
        1. Certificate of Need
    v. Oligopolies within the provider community
11. Fraud and abuse
    i. Payment system
    ii. Reimbursement
12. Excessive regulatory requirements
    i. Mandated coverage
        1. HIPAA
        2. ADA
        3. FMLA

THE SCIENTIFIC PARADIGM

Before a systems approach to healthcare outcomes management and planning can be developed and understood, one must first understand how systems work in medicine and science in general. According to Rothman in *Lessons from the Living Cell* (Rothman, 2002), "Science is seen as a rational, unbiased, or objective means of gathering and interpreting facts about nature in order to provide a clear and rigorous understanding, and eventually mastery of its properties" (Rothman, 2002, IX). Rothman continues with his description of scientific progress, "Scientific progress occurs by the sequential refinement of theories that are modified again and again, as new evidence and reason require to provide an increasingly accurate description of nature's character" (Rothman, 2002, X). Finally, Rothman describes how scientists collaborate, "As a community, scientists come to a shared sense of what is known and understood, what remains to be learned, how to learn it, and finally, what is possible and what is not" (Rothman, 2002, X). These communities of scientists share a set of assumptions about their fields of study, ones by which individual scientists define both parameters of their reality and how they investigate this reality.

At any given time, experts in a field of science tend to hold a common and comprehensive view of the system under their scrutiny. Thomas Kuhn (Kuhn, 1962) labeled this phenomenon the "paradigm." The paradigm represents a shared value judgment and belief about a particular area of study and concentration. Value judgments are rarely, if ever, the product of evidence and reason alone. Often, there is a balance between the subjective and the objective, opinion versus fact, or dogma versus theory. Kuhn noted that problems and methods outside the paradigm are denied and explained away. Science, according to Kuhn, was a social activity relying more heavily on objective analysis of data. This way, a paradigm could gain acceptance more readily than competing paradigms when it solved problems. Unfortunately, a paradigm can insulate a community of scientists from problems outside the paradigm, simply because these problems cannot be stated in terms used by those within the shared community.

Paradigms can change but not without great difficulty. In fact, according to Kuhn, paradigm shifts exhibit the following steps: awareness of anomaly, observational and conceptual recognition, and finally, change of paradigm categories and procedures (Kuhn, 1962). Resistance both within the community of scientists and outside the paradigm create a revolution of changing beliefs and values that have an incredible impact on the recipients of the change. Change in science is inevitable; Kuhn noted that criticisms of accepted values and beliefs are propagated by the young and new scientists to the field of study.

Healthcare delivery systems are no different than any other field of science whether it is basic, clinical, or applied in its categorization or classification. The key term is "system" and it is this term that leads to the discussion on how the system in health care should operate and function. Obviously, a shared set of beliefs, judgments, and values guide the healthcare delivery system in its daily activities. Commonalities among clinicians and patients, their families, and friends, keep the accepted mode of operation harmonious. This harmony results in good patient clinical outcomes and satisfaction with healthcare services received. But what is a system and how does the system in health care lend itself to the medical paradigm?

THE HEALTHCARE "SYSTEM"

What is a "system?" George Engel, MD, presented a landmark discourse (Engel, 1980) to the American Psychiatric Association's 132nd Annual Meeting, in which he described a natural or nature's "system" in the following manner:

1. Each system in nature is at the same time a component of a higher system of nature.
2. The continuity of natural systems has each unit in a system and the same time a whole and a part (i.e., an individual represents the highest level of organismic hierarchy and the lowest level of social hierarchy).
3. Each system as a whole has its own unique characteristics and dynamics; as a part it is a component of a higher level system.
4. A natural system has a stable configuration in time and space.
5. The stable configuration is maintained by coordinating the component parts of the system into an internal dynamic network while maintaining its structure as a component part of a higher level system.

6. The stable configuration of the system also implies the existence of boundaries between organized systems across which material and information will flow.
7. A natural system cannot be fully characterized as a dynamic system without characterizing the larger system of which it is a component part, (i.e., its environment).
8. Scientists that study natural systems can only focus on one system at a time to concentrate their efforts in understanding the dynamics that make that system unique from others (Engel, 1980).

The focus of study in healthcare delivery has been at the patient-clinician level. As a two-person system, the clinical encounter between a clinician and a patient represents both the highest level of the organismic system (i.e., cell, tissue, organ, organ system, patient) and the lowest level of a social system (i.e., patient, family, community, culture, society, biosphere). The healthcare delivery scientist or systems-oriented investigator identifies the constituent components of the "patient" with great precision and detail. By applying diverse and refined techniques over time, both the constituent parts of the "patient" system and how the "patient" is a component of the clinical encounter or two-person system (with the clinician) can be discovered and studied. Understanding the rules and focus responsible for the collective order of the patient-clinician system requires different approaches. The "patient-clinician" system is a component part of the healthcare delivery system. In today's study of the healthcare delivery system, adding value for the healthcare consumer, the "patient," has become the focus for much of healthcare delivery. Developing a health care delivery system that understands the systems approach to the clinical encounter requires the following:

- Improving the quality of care
- Giving consumers/patients more control over individual healthcare decisions
- Enhancing affordability
- Improving service and creating better patient experiences
- Improving access to healthcare services
- Promoting patient education
- Providing timely and accurate clinical information
- Improving convenience
- Strengthening personal relationships by improving the coordination of patient care

Engel (Engel, 1980) notes:

> "Systems-oriented physician is alerted to the possibility, if not the probability, that the course of the illness and the care of the patient may be importantly influenced by processes at the psychological and interpersonal levels of organization."

In the healthcare delivery system, actions at the biological, psychological, and social levels are dynamically interrelated and these relationships affect both the process and outcome of care. The continuum of care—from prevention to acute onset of illness to chronicity and/or recovery and remission—provides the necessary structure to identify the critical parts of the clinical encounter which result in better outcomes management of the "patient."

CHAPTER 5

The Biomedical Point of View

INTRODUCTION TO BIOMEDICINE

The history and development of the biomedical view started with the belief in the early centuries that spirits and demons were once a vital part of human existence (Longino, 1995). Life was replete with uncertainty. Over time, taming the body and life became viewed as a sign of progress. Medicine was thought to be a part of a unique cosmo. The will of gods infiltrated every aspect of peoples' lives. Mystical forces, hidden causes, and cryptic signs were commonplace. Both meditation and technical skill were necessary to produce a cure for the ill and injured. The practice of medicine was sustained by a defending god's goodness and omnipotence in view of the existence of will.

The move from the practice of religious medicine towards scientific medicine required direct observation of the patient by the clinician, logical analysis of what was observed as the cause for ill health, the dissection of nature, and a basic scientific pursuit for objective truth. Myth and speculation were to be replaced by objective fact.

Only factors that could be directly observed by the clinician were believed to help treatment. By eliminating the unknown and replacing it with observations, serious errors in the clinical practice of medicine could begin to be eliminated.

The deanimation of nature and the natural activities that surrounded life would now become real and more meaningful to both clinician and patient. The judicious reasoning process, resulting in the development of objective facts, would become the cornerstone for the medical care. Clinicians could begin to focus on their craft, and professional standards for the clinical practice of medicine could be developed. Sound clinical judgments are now based on unbiased observations which result from the accurate measurement of nature's phenomena. This lends itself to a straightforward plan of clinical action because there is objective, reliable, and valid clinical knowledge coming from an organic source.

CARTESIANISM

Rene Descartes (Longino, 1995), during the 1630s and 1640s, laid the groundwork for the scientific method, western scientific thought, and the doctrine of mind-body dualism. These three ideas became known as "Cartesianism"; this paradigm asserts that one cannot accept the unity of body and soul because they are different substances. Cartesianism believes that clinical medicine requires the mind and body to be attached because one affects the other in actual life. Living persons should be treated differently than dead persons. Therefore, dualism is not necessarily between mind and body but between clinical and scientific medicine; body with mind versus the cadaver. Medical examination of living patients should be conducted by availing oneself only of life and ordinary conversations.

The schism of mind from body led to displacement of the patient as a person. This split encouraged clinicians to examine the body as though it were still a functioning corpse, devoid of mind and spirit. The autopsy moves backwards in the process from death to cause. Correlating pathological outcomes with presumed physiological causes set the standards for study of the living. This established the accepted practice with the living for physicians to make diagnoses that could be called "autopsies in advance." As a result of attributing a damaged component to a corpse, extrapolations could be made about the manner as well as the mechanism of death. Unfortunately, this mind-body dualism became a barrier to understanding the psychosocial components of clinical medicine, the environmental components of clinical medicine, the placebo effect, the connection between stress and illness, the importance of social support for the ill patient, and the relevance of lifestyle and issues pertaining to environmental health and well-being.

Cartesianism was the early precursor to today's study and discipline of the basic medical sciences. Biologists study biological systems or bodies of living or once-living organisms. Human biology accepts the body as a biological system and avails the study of the human body to the principles of studying living systems. Therefore, technology and financial resources have been made available for studying the human body as a system and maintaining the mind-body dualism. To summarize, Zanner (Zanner, 1988) describes the "Descartes Triad" which established the true meaning behind mind-body dualism and the separation of the basic from the clinical medical sciences:

- What belongs to the mind is considered "in itself"
- What belongs to the body and to the body in general is considered "in itself" (i.e., anatomy, physiology, biochemistry, pathology) using the mechanical analogy for study of the body
- What belongs to the mind-body composite (i.e., medicine and surgery)

After Descartes, the true meaning of Cartesianism was lost and the study of the human body was replaced by the mechanical analogy in both scientific and clinical medicine.

EMPIRICISM

Clinicians became known as empiricists during the 1700s. Knowledge gained by clinicians was based on direct observation while working with patients. The data was recorded when direct observations and experimentation was performed at the bedside or in the laboratory. Little commentary was included in the reports of the physical reality observed and measured. The human "body" became a "thing of study." The human body clinically was considered transparent and simply organic material. The basis of life was identified as a collection of chemical compounds, biochemical reactions, structural components, and physiological phenomena.

The body as a "machine" dominated the philosophical approach to clinical practice during this time. This philosophy carried the study of the human body and experience from the vitalistic monism of religious practice to the materialistic monism of biomedical practice. This paradigm severed the body from the mind and thus allowed for the body's matter to be inspected completely by the clinical observer. Mind, spirit, consciousness, and soul could not compromise the pursuit for clinical knowledge.

The human body became an object that was encountered like anything else in the environment. The human body was a part of nature waiting to be probed, prodded, or rearranged. During this time, natural laws related to biochemistry and physiology were discovered and discussed amongst scientists and clinicians. Mechanization allowed for the body to break into its components or individual parts. Each component is complete and self-contained: molecules, organelles, cells, tissues, and organs.

The concept of "homeostasis" was introduced and became the leading paradigm of this time. It defined an interlocking network of causes, functions, control mechanisms, and directions the body takes biochemically and physiologically to remain in a steady state of health and well-being. The human body became available for more observation and intervention, for more examination and classification. Mechanization of the body required separation, detachment, purification, and demarcation of the human body and its components for clear perception and clarity.

Subjectivity was noted during this time to distort perception of the scientific and clinical observer and to confuse the pursuit of knowledge. Both scientists and clinicians of this time believed that subjectivity was the main source of error; it must be overcome if reliable knowledge was to be uncovered. Individual values, commitments, and personal beliefs were not allowed to invade the direct observations and measurements of biochemical and physiological phenomena. Opinions, emotions, and personal insights had no validity unless they could be tied to empirical data.

Knowledge would become power when it was purified and transformed into something universal, constant, and worthy of dissemination. Understanding the mechanization of the body resulted in the present day reliance on the technological advancements used in the diagnostic and therapeutic devices driven by modern medicine (e.g., stethoscope, oph-thalmoscope, laryngoscope, microscope, x-rays).

Biomedical science advanced over the next several years to become the modern day Western medical approach, both scientifically and clinically. Human sources of error are believed to be controlled as the clinical and laboratory setting has become systematically regulated and administered. Facts replaced opinions and data superseded individual feelings and emotions. Causes and their effects were joined in nature by material connections.

A unified theory of nature has resulted in the biomedical paradigm accepted today by many medical scientists and clinicians. "Koch's Postulates" became a prime example of cause and effect when looking for isolated etiology for disease and illness. Dubos's (Dubos, 1959) "Doctrine of Specificity" led the way for understanding biochemical lesions, molecular pathology, congenital anomalies, and genetic disorders as physical factors becoming more visible with proper preparation in the laboratory and in the clinic.

The Western medical doctrine moved beyond the mind-body dualism of Cartesianism, and accepted that the human body is to be understood as only material in nature.

WESTERN BIOMEDICAL DOCTRINE

The scientific paradigm for Western medicine is objective, reductionistic, and rational. Biomedical beliefs are based on biological and physical scientific theory and practice. Basic sciences (i.e., anatomy, physiology, biochemistry, pathology, pharmacology) and the clinical sciences (i.e., medicine, surgery, pediatrics, obstetrics and gynecology, and their subspecialties) follow the doctrine that diagnosing and treating disease located in the body is the primary purpose of their quest. Subdoctrines (Longino, 1995) within this paradigm include:

- Mind-body dualism. The mind and body are essentially different and medicine is restricted to considerations related only to the body.
- Mechanical analogy. The body is analogous to a machine and understood in terms of components creating a whole, working entity.
- Physical reductionism. Medical answers are thought to be more valid and reliable when they are founded on the basic sciences of anatomy, physiology, biochemistry, and pathology. Reductionism

attempts to understand the human body by studying its components and how they are interrelated.

- Specific etiology. A single and specific cause exists for every disease and through basic scientific methodology, each cause can be discovered and a cure provided for every illness.
- Regimen and control. A patient's physiology and biochemical activity is the proper focus of the treatment regimen and control administered by the patient's clinician (Longino, 1995, 33–51).

The mechanization of the human body reduced ambiguity and speculation on how living organisms functioned and survived. This analogy also assumes the body is standardized. However, what basic medical science has learned by studying the anatomy of the human body is that there is great variation between individuals, much like individual personalities. A well body is considered to be a fully functional machine, whereas a sick body is considered to be a broken machine. What mechanization of the human body has allowed for is a simplification process that relies on assumptions and makes the pursuit of science possible. Disease has been traditionally defined as a morbid state or process. Disease in the human body represents a condition that deviates from norms that have measurable biological parameters. The concept of "normal" or "within the normal range" is central to modern Western biomedicine. Departures from normality are diagnostic clues that the machine, or some part of it, is broken. Keeping within this paradigm, it follows that determining what is broken allows for repair of the machine and restoration back to the normal range.

The goal for biological sciences is to uncover the mechanisms of disease in organisms, use this knowledge to intervene in the disease process, and repair the machine. The goal in clinical medical sciences is to fully understand the working of the normal body and restore it to its normal functioning when broken. Reductionism enables this process to take place by establishing a paradigm of investigation for the human body and studying how each component relates from a genetic, biochemical, and pathophysiological perspective. Definitions, ideology, and exercising influence and power have a direct effect on the outcomes expected by patients, their family and friends, and clinicians. Biomedicine is bound by interpretations of fact and history, whereas cultural and social factors have no bearing on the scientific and clinical activity. Biomedicine and those that accept the paradigm attribute a "guild" mentality to the profession.

The medical establishment over the past 150 years has perpetuated the biomedical doctrine to gain political status, power, influence, and control of the healthcare delivery system. Western biomedical medicine is heaped in tradition and culture that has shaped American health care for some time. The biomedical point of view remains a very useful paradigm for the advancement of medical science today; however, strict adherence to its doctrine is very limiting and narrow in scope when applied independently of other points of view in the delivery of healthcare services.

An explanation for the biomedical paradigm that originated in the study of purely physical phenomena has been extended to biological and social phenomena (Hull, 1981). All events are explained in terms of antecedent events organized in causal chains and networks, characterized by universal laws which make no reference to the causal efficacy of future events or to higher levels of organization. Science assumes an ordered universe for otherwise the world could not be studied effectively; this includes the human body.

As a scientific strategy, reducing clinical medicine to genetic, biochemical, and pathophysiological phenomena means only that where possible, research should take a certain bend toward molecular mechanisms (Zucker, 1981). The presupposition of reduction in clinical medicine is that all disease is genetic, biochemical, and pathophysiological phenomena that has gone astray. Where there is truly no genetic, biochemical, and pathophysiological problem, there is no disease.

The ideal goal of reductionistic clinical medicine would be to have diagnostic and therapeutic interventions accomplished by performing a biophysical survey of the patient's body. Ideally, psychological, social, and environmental problems would be captured by this technique. It is part of the assumptions of reductionistic clinical medicine that, at the very least, psychosocial and environmental states have clinically useful correlations for diagnostic and therapeutic interventions.

Pure biomedical scientists look at holistic, complimentary, or alternative clinical medicine as violating the fundamental scientific understanding of causation (Longino, 1995). Ambiguity and theoretical constructs in non-Western clinical medical practice fail to satisfy the strict adherence to objective, measurable phenomena required by clinical biomedical practice. Reductionism is best supported in this paradigm of fundamental scientific understanding of causation through the pursuit of genetic determinism.

The genetic causes of disease discovered through recent work has allowed for an easy path to finding fault in the human body as a means of explaining all disease states. The use of the laboratory in mapping the human genome to discover genetic causes of disease has rekindled the focus for modern clinical medicine on the idea of the "discrete cure" for disease.

Each disease state has a unique cause that can be discovered and attacked. The germ theory and the invention of vaccines and antibiotics to attack microorganisms laid the groundwork for this paradigmatic belief used in genetic determinism today. It fits well into the scientific framework of causality being linear and concrete. Unfortunately, the laboratory—and for that matter, the hospital setting—is a very controlled environment. It potentially excludes the psychosocial and environmental aspects that the patient experiences that may contribute to the overall effects of disease.

Most disease processes involve the indirect influence of a complex set of factors—some predisposing, some precipitating and some perpetuating. Longino and Murphy (Longino, 1995) with respects to specific etiology note the following:

> As an important dimension of the biomedical model, the view that a disease has a specific cause that can be cured keeps the focus of research, diagnosis and treatment on the human body, as opposed to the contributing or participating factors outside of physiology. No one dies directly from smoking or smog, but these factors can clearly contribute to disease outcomes. And by focusing on specific etiology, attention is diverted away from issues of health promotion or disease prevention, and thus this viewpoint tends to depreciate public health approaches to industrial and environmental medicine (Longino, 1995, 47).

Western clinical biomedical practice accepts that the human body is the appropriate locus of regimen and control for eradicating genetic, biochemical, and pathophysiological disease. This is the logical corollary to the acceptance of physical reductionism; if disease is in the body, then the body would be the appropriate locus of treatment. Specific etiology is the discovery of disease or the diagnosis, and regimen and control is the treatment that follows diagnosis.

The development of the hospital as the major locus of healthcare delivery evolved as a means to isolate the patient so that clinicians could exercise control during both the diagnosis and therapeutic phases of the patient's clinical care. With patients in the hospital, the clinicians could hold other variables constant when searching for a cause and applying treatment for a disease. Moving down a decision tree to a diagnostic conclusion became easier with patients in the hospital and not out in the community.

The patient is not a passive partner in the therapeutic relationship (Longino, 1995). Emotions, perceptions, and feelings all have an effect on the outcomes of therapeutic interventions. In addition, cooperation with regimen and control requires discipline on the part of the patient. Patients must believe in the skill and power of the "healer" and the efficacy, effectiveness, and efficiency of the therapeutic intervention (e.g., allopathic care includes pharmaceuticals, procedures, and surgery).

Classifying the genetic, biochemical, and pathophysiological mechanism is easy compared to understanding how this pathogen is working in an individual, living patient who is not an isolated human body, but also has a mind and is adapted or maladapted to a complex psychosocial and physical environment (Longino, 1995).

CHAPTER 6

The Biopsychosocial Point of View

THE BIOPSYCHOSOCIAL APPROACH TO CLINICAL MEDICINE

The biomedical approach to healthcare delivery is conducive only to handling acute, rapid onset, and short-duration disease processes. There is a discrete cause of disease that can be identified and an effect can be manifested by the human body resulting in treatment and resolution of the disease process: remission, cure, or death. However, the biomedical approach is too narrow in scope to handle the complex nature of chronic disease.

Chronic diseases processes, in contrast to acute disease processes, have a slow onset, a long duration, and multiple etiologies. Chronic disease processes do not have a discrete cause and effect. Chronic disease processes, like cancer and diabetes mellitus, affect the entire human being physically, psychologically, socially, and spiritually and often have a questionable prognosis (i.e., cure, remission, or death).

Most medical treatment available in the current healthcare delivery system within the United States is complex, technology-driven, and aimed at treatment to cure, alleviate pain and suffering, restore maximum physical and psychological function, and prolong life at any cost (Longino, 1995). The future of healthcare delivery in the United States requires a paradigm shift from the curative bias of traditional Western medical dogma to an emphasis on the whole patient in three aspects: mind and body interaction, the patient and their environmental relationships, and human physiology and culture. Persons must be active in disease prevention and health promotion. The World Health Organization in 1948 (WHO, 1948) defined "Health" as the following: "Health is a state of complete physical, mental and social well-being and not merely the absence of disease or infirmity."

The structure of healthcare delivery cannot be divorced from the philosophy of Western biomedical dogma. A more complex approach to healthcare delivery is required and must be reinforced by the longstanding theories and applications of Western biomedical thought. Longino and Murphy (Longino, 1995) describe a general reorientation of Medicine that combines both a complex, all-inclusive orientation to the patient with a biomedical approach to healthcare delivery:

1. Absolutism and exclusiveness of the dualistic approach should be abandoned, along with the resulting materialism and narrow view of causality. Human life should no longer be thought to consist primarily of biophysical elements that are mechanically united.
2. Cultural, socioeconomic, political and other contextual factors must be considered in treating patient's illnesses.
3. Factors relevant to health and illness should be expanded in order to understand the nature of disease:
   a. Biogenetics
   b. Pathophysiology
   c. Psychology
   d. Sociocultural
   e. Environmental
   f. Technical
4. A new range of interventions, which were possibly dismissed as unscientific, must be explored:
   a. Complimentary and alternative care
   b. Consideration of the holistic patient (Longino, 1995)

Much of what is necessary to change the outcomes management of patient care both today and in the future does not fall traditionally within the realm sanctioned and regulated by medical professionals. What is really required is a change in the intellectual and organizational framework of the current American healthcare delivery system.

George Engel noted in 1977 (Engel, 1977) that within clinical medicine, actions at the biological, psychological, and social level are dynamically interrelated and that these relationships affect both the process and outcomes of care. He went on to note that disease and illness do not manifest themselves only in terms of biochemical changes and pathophysiology. In fact, disease and illness may simultaneously affect many different levels of functioning.

A biopsychosocial perspective involves an appreciation that disease and illness do not manifest themselves only in term of pathophysiology, biochemical change, congenital anomalies, or genetic disorders, but also may simultaneously affect many different levels of functioning, from cellular to organ system to person to family to society to biosphere. This approach provides a broader understanding of disease processes by encompassing multiple levels of functioning including the effect of the physician-patient relationship. Another approach, called the BPBETS approach, includes a more complex, inclusive categorization that builds off of what Engel started. It includes the following: biogenetic, psychological, behavioral, environmental, technical, and sociocultural areas of inquiry and will be discussed later in the chapter (see Table 6-1).

Much of Engel's comments were based on the works of biologists like Paul Weiss and Ludwig von Bertalanffy (Frankel, Quill, and McDaniel, 2003). In the systems theory of biology, a common sense approach through observation was made that nature is ordered as *hierarchically-arranged continuum*, with its more complex, larger units' super-ordinate to the less complex, smaller units. Each level in this hierarchically-arranged continuum is organized as a dynamic whole with an identity to justify its being named. The name of the level reflects the distinctive properties and characteristics that are unique and distinctive to its level. Each level requires specific criteria for study and explanation and rules of study do not apply across levels in the hierarchy. Each level (or system) is at the same time a component of a higher system. In the continuity of natural systems, every unit is at the same time both a whole and a part.

The system, on the other hand, is stable in its configuration in time and space. Boundaries exist between organized systems in nature across which information and material can flow. The system does not exist in isolation. It is maintained via coordination of its component parts in some internal

Table 6-1   BPBETS Model of Healthcare Delivery

1. Biogenetic
   a. Family history of disease
   b. Exposure to infectious agents
   c. Immunologic competence
   d. Medical history
      i. Current diseases
      ii. Surgical history
      iii. Allergies
      iv. Medications
      v. Alternative treatment
   e. Immunization history
   f. Congenital defects
   g. Impairment and disability
   h. Chronological age
   i. Growth and developmental history
   j. Gender

2. Psychological
   a. Cognitive ability
   b. Adaptability
   c. Sense of self
   d. Creativity
   e. Optimism
   f. Health locus of control
   g. Interpersonal skills
   h. Personality type
   i. Psychiatric disease
   j. Family history of mental illness

3. Behavioral
   a. Nutritional status and activity
   b. Tobacco history
   c. Alcohol consumption
   d. Illicit drug use
   e. Sleep hygiene
   f. Exercise
   g. Safety practices
      i. Seat belt wear
      ii. Helmet wear
      iii. Sexual activity
      iv. Pre-natal activity
   h. Healthy lifestyle and promotion
   i. Compliance with prescribed medical regimens

   j. Use of community resources and health services
   k. Ethical health practices
      i. Healthcare fiduciary
   l. Violence
      i. Home
      ii. School
      iii. Worksite

4. Environmental
   a. Climactic and geographic risks
      i. Earthquakes
      ii. Floods
      iii. Tornados
      iv. Temperature extremes
      v. Draught
      vi. Hurricanes
   b. Groundwater purity
      i. Soil contamination
   c. Radon exposure
   d. Ultraviolet radiation
   e. Ozone depletion
   f. Global warming
   g. Reduced biodiversity
   h. Carcinogenic exposures
   i. Air pollution
      i. Indoor
      ii. Outdoor
   j. Toxicological monitoring
      i. Physical
      ii. Chemical
      iii. Biological
   k. Natural environment and wilderness restoration

5. Technological
   a. Nontoxic construction materials
   b. Human genome
   c. Bioengineering
      i. Bionics
      ii. Prosthetics
      iii. Cloning
   d. Informatics
      i. Knowledge management
      ii. Data management

Table 6-1   BPBETS Model of Health Care Delivery *(continued)*

iii. Internet technology
iv. Web-based access
e. Ergonomic design
f. Environmental aesthetics
g. Engineering safety
   i. Power vehicles
   ii. Noise
   iii. Electromagnetic radiation
   iv. Water quality
   v. Sanitation

6. Sociocultural
  a. Socioeconomic status
   i. Individual
   ii. Population
  b. Social support
   i. Customs
   ii. Bereavement
   iii. Friendship
  c. Religious and spiritual beliefs
  d. Political structure
   i. Regulation
   ii. Legislation
   iii. Administration
   iv. Local, regional, state, national, global
  e. Economics
   i. Microeconomics
    A. Supply
    B. Demand

   ii. Macroeconomics
    A. Employment
    B. Taxation
    C. Inflation
  f. Communication
   i. Interpersonal
   ii. Media
  g. Population health management
   i. Health enhancement
   ii. Risk assessment
   iii. Disease management
   iv. Demand management
   v. Disability management
  h. Insurability
   i. Health
   ii. Life
   iii. Disability
   iv. Long term care
   v. Ancillary services
   vi. Mental health
   vii. Worker's compensation
  i. Accessibility to health care
   i. Legislation
   ii. Regulation
   iii. Administration
  j. Healthcare finance
   i. Cost benefit analysis
   ii. Spending
   iii. Funding
    A. Private
    B. Public

dynamic network. It also has characteristics and constituents of a larger system of which it is a component. The system can be influenced by the configuration of the systems of which each is a part (i.e., its environment).

Engel (Engel, 1980) was instrumental in developing an approach with two hierarchies:

- An organismic hierarchy defining the individual person at the highest level of this system. Subatomic particles—Atoms—Molecules—Organelles—Cells—Tissues—Organs—Organ Systems—Nervous system—Person. The individual person brings experience and behavior to the highest point of this hierarchy and is also the lowest component of the next hierarchical system.

- A social hierarchy defining the population as a whole with the community at the highest level of this system. Person—Two person—Family—Community—Culture/Subculture—Society/Nation—Biosphere.

Health care chooses to begin efforts of scientific investigation at the system level identified as the "person." A systems-oriented clinical investigator in classical Western Biomedical approach identifies the constituent components of the "person" system and characterizes each component in great detail with precise accuracy. Over time, this clinical investigation must apply increasingly diverse and refined techniques to extend knowledge about constituent parts of the system. In addition, the system's characteristics of each component part of the "person" system must also be studied.

Different approaches are required to gain understanding of the rules and focus responsible for the collective order of this system. The system-oriented investigator must keep in mind the hierarchically-oriented continuum concept. The classic biomedical investigator who studies the "person" system in Western medicine has the ultimate explanatory power of the factor-analytic approach which, in effect, inhibits attention to what characterizes the whole system.

Engel wrote (Engel, 1980) that Western biomedical approaches neglect the whole inherent concept in the reductionistic model of biomedicine. This, he believed, was largely responsible for the physician pre-occupation with the body alone and with disease and the corresponding neglect of the patient as a whole. According to Engel, the disease process simultaneously encompasses multiple levels of functioning, including the effect of the physician-patient relationship (e.g., a two-person component of a social hierarchy).

A comprehensive understanding of every aspect of healthcare delivery—from diagnosis to treatment—depends on appreciating a system of both linear and non-linear processes associated with disease and illness. It is the culture of the social hierarchy and how the individual person assimilates into that culture that requires an understanding of interpersonal and sociocultural phenomenon for conceptualizing disease and illness. The essence of what Engel proposed leads into the importance of understanding the success of clinicians. These clinicians are able to incorporate knowledge about the effects of culture in a social hierarchical continuum. This group of clinicians also applies the approach to the symptoms present in individual patients. These clinicians are more likely to accurately understand and treat their patients, resulting in higher quality of care and improved outcomes.

The biopsychosocial approach requires that a human being be viewed as a biological organism and the highest level of a hierarchical system, as well as a person who lives in the context of family and community and the lowest level of another hierarchical system. Basic science, clinical research, and applied medical study has developed around this biopsychosocial approach, and has resulted in the documentation of positive biological, psychological, social, technical, and environmental outcomes.

To summarize, Engel (Engel, 1977) discussed how systems theory conforms to his biopsychosocial approach to clinical care:

> Systems theory holds that all levels of organization are linked to each other in hierarchical relationship so that change in one affects change in the others . . . for medicine, system theory provides a conceptual approach suitable not for the proposed biopsychosocial concept of disease but also for studying disease and medical care as interrelated processes . . . each system implies qualities and relationships distinctive for that level of organization, and each requires criteria for study and explanation unique for that level. In no way can the methods and rules appropriate for the study and understanding of the cell as cell be applied to the study of the family as the family.

Engel reinforces his approach in clinical medicine by stating that clinical study begins at the individual person level and takes place within a two-person system, the clinician–patient relationship, also known as the therapeutic dyad. This concept is further discussed in a later chapter.

To establish the importance of the biopsychosocial approach, social science has accepted much of what Engel proposed and places the biopsychosocial approach in the broader context of scientific discovery and advance (Frankel, Quill, and McDaniel, 2003). An important paradigm shift has occurred as acceptance for this approach has gained. According to Kuhn (Kuhn, 1962), "Paradigms are universally recognized scientific achievements (in a given field) that for a time provide model problems and solutions for a community of practitioners." A paradigm shift occurs when one or a group of scientists come to see the same facts or problems in a different light. There are two basic changes in science that are recognized theoretically—evolutionary and revolutionary change. Evolutionary change can be characterized by the following:

- Incremental in scope
- Knowledge accumulates slowly over time
- Society is often surprised by the change
- Change is normative in that it does *not* challenge methods technology, or canons of evidence or institutional frameworks
- It has intellectual and not institutional effects (Frankel, Quill, and McDaniel, 2003)

Revolutionary change, on the other hand, can be characterized by the following:

- An entire system of thought is questioned by new knowledge or thinking
- Fundamental assumptions in a scientific field are challenged
- Change often gives rise to a new scientific field of study
- It has both intellectual and institutional effects (e.g., the discovery of DNA led to the new scientific field of molecular biology)
- There is a rapid and complete change (Frankel, Quill, and McDaniel, 2003).

The question has arisen over the last several decades between current Western biomedical approach proponents and the biopsychosocial approach proponents as to whether a true paradigmatic shift has occurred in clinical medicine regarding the development of a new field of study using the biopsychosocial approach. Interestingly, there has been an incomplete shift with limited results.

Current biomedical proponents have met the biopsychosocial proponents with hostility and intense disdain. Even so, there are many that believe that the biopsychosocial approach supplements and enriches the discoveries that are being made in biomedical circles of scientific thought. There remains a lack of consensus around a common conceptualization. There is a gap between the qualities of experience that individual patients and clinicians bring to the therapeutic dyad (a two-person system) at any given time and place. However, it is the population perspective, not the individual patient experience, that lies at the heart of current understanding of incidence and prevalence of disease (Frankel, Quill, and McDaniel, 2003).

Disease and risk factors are meaningful and predictable in relationship to the entire population. Prediction occurs not at the level of the individual uncertainty but in terms of probability. There is a tension that remains between individual patient knowledge and the knowledge gained and accepted within the scientific community. There is also a tension that remains between qualitative and quantitative analysis methodologies in scientific exploration.

A model is a belief system used to explained natural phenomena. A scientific model is a shared set of assumptions and rules of conduct based on the scientific methods and constitutes a blueprint for research and scientific inquiry. Social science research and qualitative analysis adds depth of knowledge to the quantitative data obtained through vigorous scientific study. Qualitative analysis also helps to interpret quantitative findings, generates hypotheses for future exploration, and explores the exceptions to the scientific rule.

The biopsychosocial approach is really a "folk" model of qualitative analysis employing a culturally derived belief system that promotes social adaptation. As later discussed in the text, outcomes management and planning serves as the glue both conceptually and methodologically for using the biomedical and biopsychosocial approach in a complimentary manner to explore individuals and populations with illness and disease.

CLINICAL PRACTICE AND THE BIOPSYCHOSOCIAL APPROACH

The biopsychosocial approach initiated a paradigm shift in Western biomedical thought by recognizing that considering only structural, biochemical, and physiological aspects of a human being was insufficient to explain illness and suffering (Epstein et al., 2003). The biopsychosocial approach makes clear distinction between suffering, illness, and disease. Disease represents a structural alteration or measurable physiologic malfunctioning. Illness accepts that human beings are more than unfortunate hosts of pathophysiology. Illness includes the subjective sense of being unwell, as well as the effect that the disease process has on the patient as a person and as a member of a social community. Epstein points out that disease can exist in the absence of illness (e.g., asymptomatic state), illness can exist in the absence of disease (e.g., psychogenic pain syndrome), and suffering can exist in the absence of both disease and illness. Suffering is contextual and relates to a patient's beliefs, family background, sociodemographic status, gender, education, access to care, etc.

Epstein provides a complete spectrum of the central aspects of the biopsychosocial approach including eliciting the patient's story and life circumstances, integrating the biological, psychological, social, and environmental domains, recognizing the centrality of relationships in providing healthcare services, understanding the healthcare provider, focusing the biopsychosocial approach for clinical practice, and providing multidimensional treatment for the individual patient that can be applied to populations or subpopulations.

The biopsychosocial approach differs from traditional Western biomedical thought in that it allows for multifactorial causation to explore the biological, psychological, and social ramifications of all illness (Engel, 1988). The real focus of this approach encompasses healthcare delivery in relationship to the patient and the system. The biopsychosocial approach does not advocate any one particular clinical method or treatment. It is not alternative or complimentary care. The scope of clinical practice may at times be narrowly circumscribed and apply a singular causal model for all illness if necessary.

The biopsychosocial approach is not exclusive to primary care medicine. All specialties in clinical medicine benefit from fostering effective patient communication; understanding the patient's perspective on disease, illness, and suffering; understanding psychosocial determinants of health; and exercising shared decision making. This approach focuses better on issues important to both clinician and patient, and results in more effective and efficient healthcare delivery (Stewart et al., 2000). The complexity of a medical case can be compartmentalized into smaller amounts of data and information. This organizes important clinical data for incremental application of a multidimensional clinical approach that increases the probability of improved outcomes for both the patient and the clinician.

ELICITING THE PATIENT'S STORY AND LIFE CIRCUMSTANCES

Epstein describes the illness narrative as the patient's spontaneous expression of a story on his or her terms (Epstein et al., 2003). The clinician must exercise patience and understanding while allowing the patient to describe his/her issues with minimal intrusion by the clinician. The clinician's skill and experience in practicing this process helps to gain the patient's trust so that his/her story can be explored in a fuller context, including family and culture, followed by an active diagnostic inquiry of symptoms using the biomedical approach. The elements of the symptom presentation include the verbal exchange between the patient and the clinician, non-verbal communication between the patient and the clinician, contextual features (see Table 6-2) interpreted from the patient's perspective, and the time allotted by the clinician to elicit the patient's story.

Outcomes management and planning are related to the degree to which patients and clinicians agree on the nature of the patient's presenting complaint. Outcomes are also related to the degree to which the patient feels understood and empowered to have an active role in his/her care. The biopsychosocial aspects of a patient's life must take into consideration the human contextual features of the patient's illness experience. According to research in this area (Stewart et al., 1997), understanding the patient's story improves three outcomes in a managed care environment: clinical performance, patient satisfaction, and cost.

Table 6-2   Patient's Contextual Features

1. Individual history
2. Individual beliefs
3. Family background
4. Socioeconomic status
5. Educational background
6. Likes and dislikes
7. Values
8. Ethnicity
9. Gender
10. Access to healthcare services
11. Community
12. Geography

Table created from material in Epstein, RM, Morse, DS, Williams, GC, leRoux, P, Suchman, AL, Quill, TE. Clinical practice and the biopsychosocial approach. In: Frankel, RM, Quill, TE, McDaniel, SH eds. The biopsychosocial approach: past, present, and future. Rochester, NY: University of Rochester Press 2003. 33–66.

INTEGRATING BIOLOGICAL, PSYCHOLOGICAL, SOCIAL, AND ENVIRONMENTAL DOMAINS

The biopsychosocial approach uses the tools of evidence-based medicine, epidemiology, and population medicine to allow for the expansion of relevant information from the patient's psychological and social domains. Patient emotions, family dynamics, culture, and economics may also come into use because they can affect medical decision making. Strong epidemiologic data (Epstein et al., 2003) link depression, anxiety, and somatization in the primary care setting to presenting complaints of fatigue, palpitations, and chronic pains. Research suggests that primary care clinicians fail to use these tools to recognize mental disorders on a regular basis (i.e., depression, bipolar disorders) and the narrow use of biomedical workups for suggestive symptoms are the norm (Escobar, 1996; Coyne, 1994).

Epstein acknowledges (Epstein et al., 2003) that a fundamental tension exists between strict biomedical thinking and biopsychosocial thinking. A patient's illness experience is unique to them. Diagnostic categories, on the other hand, are attempts to abstract and categorize illness experiences into discrete disease entities. The diagnostic schema of twentieth century Western biomedical medicine is powerful and predictive and provides a link between symptoms, signs, and pathophysiological mechanisms affecting both mind and body. On the other hand, personal, social, and family aspects of illness are often idiosyncratic; although patterns of family and social relations exist, each family is unique. It is this uniqueness that leads the biopsychosocial approach to the forefront of modern medicine today, and enables it to assist the biomedical approach in developing a comprehensive diagnosis of a patient's problems with the following categories: pathophysiological abnormalities, biochemical change, structural abnormalities, genetic disorders, psychosocial descriptors, and environmental exposures.

Acceptable outcomes lead the clinician today to perform three simultaneous tasks when caring for patients: gathering adequate descriptions of the patient's symptoms to arrive at a diagnosis of disease processes, knowing enough about the patient's inner experiences to understand the meaning of the illness, and observing patterns of personal and social relationships to understand the fabric of the patient's life.

CENTRALITY OF RELATIONSHIPS IN PROVIDING HEALTHCARE SERVICES

The quality of the relationship that develops between a clinician and the patient may have a direct effect upon outcomes management. The patient's well-being, the patient's satisfaction with the delivery of health services, and the principal determinant of clinician satisfaction (e.g., personal, economic, or professional satisfaction) are three main areas affected by this relationship. The clinician always has an unfair advantage over the patient in this relationship. Professional power resulting from education and training must be used judiciously in a fiduciary manner so as to responsibly help the patient in all facets of care. Patients should be assisted by their clinician to actively participate in all areas of their health care. The clinician must function as a coach and advisor when helping the patient discern what health issues need to be addressed and at what time. Priorities and goals for care must be established to promote healing, relieve suffering, and encourage healthy behavior (Cassel, 1982). To achieve these goals, the clinician must understand the patient biogenetically, psychologically, behaviorally, and socioculturally.

The patient needs to be understood within the context of his/her environmental surroundings. The technology now available allows this to be done effectively and efficiently. More recently, the patient-centered model has emerged as one of the more accepted methods of reaching a strong patient–clinician relationship (Epstein, 1996). In this model, the clinician and patient find the common ground on which to base medical decisions. In fact, the decision making process requires that illness be understood from the patient's perspective as well as from a diagnostic perspective. The clinician is under a moral obligation to share power with the patient and to show a human face with empathy and kindness. The patient needs to be asked how much he/she wants to participate in his/her care. Family and friends are also an important constituent and must be included in the discussion of care when treating patients using this model.

Patients have more motivation when clinicians support their needs for autonomy, competence, and relationship (Epstein et al., 2003). Autonomy implies a self determination that leaves the patient feeling that the decision he/she has made has come from within as opposed to feeling controlled or coerced by others. Patients must also feel that they possess the skills to change behavior to healthy behaviors. This feeling of competency allows for shared decision making and leads to better outcomes because both the clinician and the patient accept a mutual goal of care. Relationships that foster autonomy and competence enhance motivation and increase the patient's likelihood of maintaining long-term change with better clinical outcomes.

UNDERSTANDING THE CLINICIAN

Epstein (Epstein et al., 2003) describes in great detail the basis for the understanding the clinician:

> The most important diagnostic and therapeutic tool is the physician. A "mindful" practitioner can understand the thoughts and feelings that affect his or her own actions, and modify his or her approach based on that insight. Practicing mindfully means being attentive and present to one's own thoughts, judgments, feelings and reactions to everyday practice. Mindful practice applies equally to cognitive, emotional and technical domains. Awareness of bias is fundamental to medical decision-making and awareness of one's own clinical judgment process is fundamental to teaching others to be good clinicians. These cognitive processes can be as tacit and unconscious as emotional processes. Similarly, technical skills require self-awareness and self monitoring. The skilled surgeon maintains a level of awareness to anticipate errors in technique and judgment. Mindfulness can be learned and taught.

Clinicians will at times experience great swings in emotions as they care for patients. Certain patient behaviors can elicit emotions that can affect the therapeutic relationship. Being cognizant of this possibility and learning to control one's emotions is paramount to preserving the sanctity of the clinician–patient relationship. Recusing oneself from this relationship is sometimes necessary when a clinician's emotions cannot be held in check. Dissolving the therapeutic relationship is difficult at best and must be handled with decorum and skill. Lack of communication is the main reason for failures in the therapeutic relationship between clinician and patient. Communication is key for outcomes management, and good communication often decreases demands on the healthcare delivery system, decreases requests for specialty consultation, and reduces malpractice litigation (Lin et al., 1991; Stewart et al., 1997; Beckman et al., 1994).

FOCUS THE APPROACH FOR CLINICAL PRACTICE

The biopsychosocial approach expands the information to be gathered from the patient, family and friends; the scope of responsibility for the clinician; and the overall complexity of problem-solving (Epstein et al., 2003). Problems are seen as interacting, multidimensional, dynamic, and non-linear. In contrast, focusing on single problems, attending to disease to the exclusion of illness, and ignoring the other factors outside of the biogenetic realm when tending to patient care may seem easier to the busy clinician. Clinicians are known to pride themselves on being skilled, knowledgeable, competent, autonomous, and hard-working. A situation where uncertainty prevails creates great angst for many clinicians. Active management, shared decision-making, and collaboration amongst colleagues' results in reducing the complexity of clinical cases to more manageable, focused entities for both patient and clinician.

PROVIDING MULTIDIMENSIONAL TREATMENT

Complex case management presents the clinician with clinical management issues commonly encountered in many illnesses. The complex clinical management issues include the balance between palliative and curative healthcare delivery, the clinician and patient attitudes towards prescription drugs and medical technology for diagnostics and treatment, and medical decision making in the face of clinical uncertainty. Multidimensional treatment requires the clinician to use all available diagnostics and therapeutics so as to arrive at a mutually satisfactory treatment plan for the patient. The clinician is forced to understand the patient's degree of tolerance for uncertainty, and the risks of both not treating and of treatment. Medical decision making is influenced by family and friends, economics, and the likelihood that the patient will follow through with the clinician's recommendations for care. The human connection between physician and patient is the central ingredient in clinical care.

Epstein (Epstein et al., 2003) describes this process in the context of healing and the biopsychosocial approach:

Healing has more to do with making persons feel well and whole, and may or may not involve curing disease. Physicians can care for patients more effectively when they care about their patients in this personal way. Cures can be affected sometimes with the most minimal human interactions, but patients need to be understood to feel healed. A fundamental of biopsychosocial care is that all patients can be healed to some degree, even if they cannot be cured. The capacity to heal requires training, experience, and a facilitating environment. Patients' journeys through health and illness are often not predictable. Clinicians who have the skills and willingness to accompany their patients on these complex journeys will be more effective as healers and more satisfied with their work.

THE FUTURE OF CLINICAL BIOPSYCHOSOCIAL PRACTICE

As the biopsychosocial approach has become more accepted over time, the patient has become a multifaceted organism instead of a collection of bodily functions. Understanding this multifaceted organism by linking the biogenetic with the psychosocial has led to a progressive movement to include the patient, their family, and friends into the inner sanctum of healthcare delivery that was once protected by clinical professionalism and arrogance.

With the trend in traditional biomedical circles to specialize and fragment healthcare delivery even more than what the United States has seen over the past 30 to 40 years, clinical practice must be balanced by increasing communication, teamwork, and collaboration between the many disciplines in medicine so as to strive for improved outcomes and higher quality, more cost-effective care. Epstein (Epstein et al., 2003) describes the secrets of clinical care possessing these three qualities: curiosity, caring, and presence. It is the presence of biopsychosocially trained clinicians who are eager to apply scientific principles to the study of patients and their illness that will supply the healthcare community with enough new information to shift the paradigm toward a biopsychosocial approach that functions on an even basis with traditional biomedical theories and principles. It is this coexistence between both bodies of knowledge that will change the delivery of healthcare services to be more mindful and caring for the patients, their families, and friends.

CHAPTER 7

Applied Healthcare Outcomes Management— A Primer on Epidemiology

INTRODUCTION TO EPIDEMIOLOGY

Epidemiology is the study of the distribution and determinants of health states and disease in specified populations. There are four levels at which the scientific study of disease can be approached. The first is at the submolecular and molecular level and includes the disciplines of cell biology, genetics, biochemistry, and immunology. The second level is at the tissue and organ level and includes the disciplines of anatomy, physiology, microbiology, pharmacology, and pathology. The third level is at the individual patient level and includes the disciplines of all clinical medicine: pediatrics, surgery, internal medicine, obstetrics and gynecology, and their subspecialties. The final level is at the population level and includes the basic sciences of public health, including epidemiology and the applied medical sciences including medical ethics, health economics, medical anthropology, medical sociology, and medical psychology. Coordination of education, research, and service among all four levels is key for understanding how health and disease are interrelated. Then, the impact each has on functionality and quality of life at both the population and individual level can be measured.

AREAS OF CONCENTRATION

Jekel, Elmore, and Katz (Jekel et al., 1996) categorize epidemiology into the following areas: classical epidemiology, clinical epidemiology, infectious disease epidemiology, and chronic disease epidemiology.

Classical epidemiology is population-oriented and studies the community origins of health problems related to nutrition, the environment, human behavior, and the psychological, social, and spiritual state of a population. Classical epidemiologists are interested in discovering risk factors that might be altered in a population to prevent or delay disease or death.

Clinical epidemiology is scientifically oriented in the same way that classical epidemiology functions, and uses similar research designs and statistical tools. However, clinical epidemiology studies patients in the healthcare delivery system to improve the diagnosis, treatment, and outcomes of various disease states. Adjusting for the presence of two or more diseases and for any clinical intervention required by the patient allows for clinical epidemiology to study the delivery of clinical care and report on the outcomes derived by patients within the healthcare delivery system. This area of specialization within the study of disease can be classified as decision support analysis and more recently has been adapted to medical informatics.

Infectious disease epidemiology focuses on the laboratory analysis of microbes (e.g., bacteria, fungi, parasites, viruses, arthropods, etc.) and their impact on the development and distribution of disease in the population. This area is oriented toward public health intervention and its findings improve the health and well-being of populations through immunization programs, environmental health management, and cultural change.

Chronic disease epidemiology is a subspecialty of clinical epidemiology and focuses its attention on complex sampling and statistical methods that provide information on how to improve on the outcomes of chronic diseases (e.g., hypertension, diabetes mellitus, asthma, etc.). In this area of study, epidemiologists use the following areas of concentration to fully study the causes of the chronic disease and to provide strategies to the population for prevention: biologic factors, behavioral factors, environmental factors, immunologic factors, nutritional factors, genetic factors, social factors, spiritual factors, and service delivery factors.

NATURAL HISTORY OF DISEASE

The natural history of disease is described by categorizing the causative factors into four categories: the host, the agent, the vector, and the environment (Jekel et al., 1996). Host factors are responsible for the degree to which the individual can adapt to stressors produced by agents. Nutritional status, genotype, immune status, and social behavior collectively establish the individual's resistance to disease and an overall sense of well-being.

The agents of disease can be broken into several categories: biological, chemical, physical, social, and psychological stressors. Biological agents include all types of microbes and infectious organisms, allergens, vaccines, and foods. Chemical agents include toxins such as heavy metals, solvents, and dusts. Physical agents include kinetic energy such as blunt force trauma and firearm wounds, radiation, heat, cold, and noise. Social and psychological stressors include the effects of war, poverty, and political struggles that may reduce the individual's ability to maintain a sense of well-being.

Vectors serve as an intermediary so the agent can survive environmental challenges to get the agents of disease into direct contact with the individual. Insects, arthropods, and animals classically have been considered vectors for diseases that affect man. However, humans can also serve as vectors for agents of disease, which lead to addictions and opportunities for disease (i.e., illicit drug suppliers provide individuals with agents such as cocaine, heroin, etc.). To be an effective transmitter of disease, the vector must have a specific relationship to the agent, the environment, and the host.

The environment influences the probability and circumstances of contact between the host and the agents. Social, political, and economic factors all contribute to the environmental possibilities that engage the individual with the etiologic agents of disease. Poor economic conditions may lead to a decrease in standards of living for a population that in turn leads to poor living conditions and more susceptibility to disease.

According to Jekel et al. (1996), epidemiology is concerned with human ecology and in particular with the impact that health interventions have on the distribution of disease and on the environment. Knowing that the solution of one problem tends to create new problems, epidemiology often tries to identify the undesirable side effects of medical and public health interventions.

The principles of epidemiology include describing the health of populations, detecting causes of health problems, quantifying the association between ill health and risk factors, testing treatments and public health interventions, and monitoring changes in states of health over time. Epidemiologists contribute to the applied medical sciences by:

- Investigating the modes of transmission of a new disease
- Determining preventable causes of disease and / or injury
- Determining the natural history of disease
- Studying the biologic spectrum of disease
- Evaluating community health interventions
- Setting disease control priorities
- Improving the diagnosis, treatment, and prognosis of clinical disease
- Improving health services research
- Providing expert testimony in the medicolegal arena

EPIDEMIOLOGIC METHODOLOGY

Epidemiologic methods are often the first scientific methods applied to define a new health problem's pattern in the population and to develop hypotheses about its causes and methods of transmission. Methods of application to the control of health problems in populations can be either descriptive or analytical. There is an existence and extent of correlations between the distribution of disease and well-being, the agents which may affect this distribution, and the degree of exposure between environmental influences and the biopsychosocial characteristics of individuals in the population.

Epidemiology uses data management and basic measurements in a unique, logical framework to describe populations. Each type of epidemiologic study is especially appropriate for the unique circumstances surrounding any particular investigation of a population—the aims of the investigation, the population of persons available to study, and the human and financial resources available to study the problem at hand.

According to Friedman (2004), understanding the cause of disease and developing appropriate therapies to treat the disease involves studies of relationships of one type of event, characteristic, or variable to another. In epidemiology, the relationship most often studied is between exposure and disease. Exposure includes any of a subject's attributes or any agent with whom he or she may have been directly or indirectly in contact with that may be relevant to that subject's health and well-being. Multiple exposures are often the rule in epidemiologic investigations and the scientist must define the variables and realize how each variable relates as an exposure for the disease state in question.

There are two basic approaches to investigating the relationship between variables—observational and/or experimental studies. Observational studies allow nature to run its course. Changes or differences in one characteristic are studied in relation to changes or differences in the other, if any. Experimental studies allow for the investigator to directly intervene and make one variable change to study what effect this change has on other variables of interest. The investigator tries to prevent other important variables from affecting the outcome so that appropriate conclusions about the effect of the intervention can be made.

Observational studies fall into two main categories—descriptive and analytic. There are two fundamental objectives of observational epidemiological studies. The first objective is to describe the occurrence of disease or disease-related phenomena in populations. The second objective is to explain the observed pattern of occurrences of disease. To accomplish the second objective, causal or etiologic factors of the disease being studied must be identified.

Descriptive studies involve the determination of the incidence, prevalence, and mortality rates for diseases in populations based on basic group characteristics such as gender, ethnicity, age, and other sociodemographic factors. Then, the general distribution of disease in the population can be studied. Analytic studies attempt to explain disease occurrence in a population being studied. The starting point of any analytic study is often a descriptive finding that raises certain questions or suggests certain hypotheses requiring ongoing investigation. Analytic studies require the investigator to answer specific questions or groups of questions related to the occurrence of disease. While descriptive studies may provide large amounts of data that give a clear answer to a specific question about a population, analytic studies designed to answer a specific question may produce large amounts of descriptive data and provide an opportunity to raise further questions for investigation. Another way to differentiate between descriptive and analytic epidemiologic studies is to note that descriptive studies involve a more diffuse, superficial, or general view of a disease problem whereas analytic studies narrow to a specific question and may require a more rigorous study design and data analysis (Friedman, 2004).

Cross-sectional or prevalence studies examine the relationship between diseases and other characteristics or variables of interest as they exist in a defined population at a particular time. The presence or absence of disease and the presence or absence of other variables is determined in each member of the study population or in a representative sample. The relationship between the disease and the variable can be analyzed in two ways: either (1) in terms of the prevalence of disease in different population subgroups defined according to the presence or absence of the variable, or conversely, (2) in terms of the presence or absence of the variables in the disease versus the control population group without the disease (Friedman, 2004).

Cohort or incidence studies look more directly at attributes or factors related to the development of a disease. A study population free of the disease under investigation is identified at a particular point in time. The attributes of interest are measured initially in this group of persons known as the "cohort." Then these persons are followed over a specified period of time and are monitored for the development of the disease being studied. The relationship of an attribute to the disease is examined by dividing the population into subgroups according to the presence or absence of the attribute initially and comparing the subsequent incidence of disease in each subgroup. Cohort studies are prospective in nature because these studies involve the collection of observations after the investigation has been initiated. The prospective nature of cohort studies allows for the investigator to plan and control the scientific methodology to make and record observations (Friedman, 2004).

Case-control studies begin by initially identifying cases or persons with the disease of interest and then by identifying a suitable control group of persons without the disease being studied. The relationship of an attribute to the disease is examined by comparing the diseased and nondiseased with regard to how frequently the attribute is present or if the study is quantitative in nature, to the levels of the attribute in the two groups. Case-control studies can be similar to cross-sectional or prevalence studies if they assess the relationship of existing disease to other variables or attributes. Case-control studies can be similar to cohort or incidence studies if they assess only newly diagnosed cases. Case-control studies are retrospective in nature and use observations that have been recorded in the past. The retrospective nature of case-control studies attempt to measure past characteristics in persons with the disease already under investigation. In this context, the data recorded may well have been collected for an entirely unrelated purpose, resulting in incomplete and inappropriate data for the desired study. However, with retrospective studies all data collected may have great value and lead to a better understanding of the disease under investigation (Friedman, 2004).

BASIC EPIDEMIOLOGIC MEASUREMENT

According to Friedman (2004), epidemiology is a quantitative science. Its measured quantities and descriptive terms are used to characterize groups of persons. The simplest and most frequently performed quantitative measurement in epidemiology is a *count* of the number of persons within the studied group who have a particular disease or particular characteristic under investigation. For a count to be descriptive of a group it must be converted to a *proportion*—it must be divided by the total number in the group of persons being studied. A percentage is established and creates one of the most basic ways to describe a population. One central concern of epidemiology according to Friedman (2004) is to find and enumerate appropriate denominators to describe and compare groups of persons in a meaningful and useful way. Certain proportions, often called *rates*, are used frequently in epidemiological studies. They usually imply or involve a time relationship. The two most commonly used proportions or rates used in epidemiology are *prevalence* and *incidence*.

Prevalence, from an epidemiologic perspective, describes a group of persons at a certain point in time. It is the proportion of the number of persons with a disease divided by the total number in the group being studied at a particular point in time. It is like a snapshot of an existing situation. Incidence describes the rate at which a disease develops in a group of persons over a period of time. Compared to prevalence, incidence describes the continuing occurrence of new cases of a disease. Not everyone in a study population may be at risk for developing a disease. Often, persons already suffering from a chronic disease are removed from the denominator population under investigation because they are not at risk for the disease. *Cumulative incidence* is the proportion of a group of persons that develop a disease over a specified period of time, often long periods of time such as years. *Incidence rate* (also known as the incidence density or the hazard rate) is based on the perspective that disease may develop as a continuous process that can be described as a rate of change at any instant of time, also known as person-time. Person-time is the sum of the observation periods at risk for all persons in study group. It is usually expressed as person-years. It is another way of expressing the fact that incidence rates have both persons at risk and time in the denominator.

From an outcomes management and planning perspective, epidemiology relies on *mortality rates* to describe the process of dying. It may be expressed either as an instantaneous rate or as cumulative mortality. *Age-specific mortality rates* describe the number of persons dying in a particular age group, and is divided by the person-time in the same age group. *Case fatality rate* refers to the proportion of persons who die from the particular disease under investigation. *Proportional mortality* is simply the proportion of all deaths that are due to a particular cause. It is used when the living population at risk for the observed deaths cannot readily be enumerated, in the hope that a high proportional mortality rate for a particular disease reflects a high true mortality rate for that disease.

EPIDEMIOLOGICAL OBSERVATIONS

To describe and explain the occurrence of disease in populations, epidemiology uses a wide variety of observations and measurements (Friedman, 2004). Many factors influence human health and disease including biogenetics, pathophysiology, psychology, sociocultural, environmental, and technical factors.

In order to fully appreciate the importance of outcomes management and planning, the nature and limitations of data sources must be discussed in the context of science, scientific methodology, and everyday clinical patient healthcare delivery. All observations and measures involve some degree of error. Errors affect two important aspects of data quality—*validity* and *reliability*. Validity, or accuracy, is a measure of how closely the observations correspond to the actual state of affairs. Reliability, or reproducibility, is a measure of how closely a series of observations or measurements of exactly the same thing coincide with one another. Observations and measurements may be highly reliable but invalid. However, the lack of validity does not necessarily rule out the use of the data. If observations and measurements are unreliable, chances are these data are also invalid, and therefore not useful as true values.

Reliability is often measured in terms of the coefficient of variation for quantitative variables. This is simply the standard deviation of the set of repeated measurements used to estimate reliability divided by their average or mean, often expressed as a percentage. According to Friedman (2004), although the standard deviation itself is a measure of variability, it is put into better perspective by relating it to the average measurement because the larger the measured values, the more absolute variability is to be expected. For qualitative variables, epidemiology often uses the Kappa coefficient established by Cohen in 1960 as the index of reliability. This measure shows how much more agreement there is between variables than would be expected by chance alone. Kappa is good to use when more than one rater is evaluating the values in a study.

There are common sources of variation among data observed or measured that can not be attributed to validity or reliability. Differences among subgroups in a population, differences among individuals within the subgroup, and differences within each individual owing to a variety of influences (e.g., BPBETS model discussed in Chapter 6) appear to vary because of human or mechanical failings of the observer (Friedman, 2004).

Another source of error in observed or measured data is called *sampling variation,* and is due to chance (Friedman, 2004). It can be overcome by studying sufficiently large groups in the population. Experience in epidemiology and the laws of probability provide the explanation for choosing large samples of persons in order to discover findings that will be more representative of the total population being investigated. If repeated sampling from a population is performed, the findings in each sample subgroup will differ from one another, thus the term sampling variation. The larger the sample size studied, the less the variation and the less chance of error that can occur.

Epidemiology employs statistical significance tests (e.g., t- or chi-square tests) to measure the probability of chance errors, given the size and characteristics of the study population and the question(s) being asked. The result of a statistical significance test is a probability level or p value, commonly used in the medical literature today. The expression $p<0.05$ means that there is less than a 5 percent probability that the observed result could have occurred by chance error alone. Sampling variation can be measured using *confidence intervals* or *confidence limits.* The confidence interval or limits around a measurement or value indicate the range of values that probably contain the true value being sought within the population under investigation.

Clinical observations and measurements determine the presence or absence of a particular healthy or disease state in the population under investigation. Traditionally, medicine was forced to perfect the art of the history and physical examination of patients to generate a list of possible diagnoses. The history of the presenting complaint was elicited from the patient using the Socratic method of questioning. Symptoms that were confirmed positive or negative by the patient prompted further questioning by the examining physician until a general picture of the patients subjective concerns was developed. This was followed by a focused physical examination of the body to look for signs that confirmed the subjective symptoms established during the patient interview. Over 90 percent of all diagnoses can be determined by a skilled physician using the focused history and physical examination of patient.

Until the recent (last 60 years) advent of laboratory, radiological, and diagnostic studies, it was the history and physical examination that began the process of establishing clinical observations, and led to the differential diagnosis of disease states. From this, treatment protocols and procedures were established for patient care at the bedside. Essentially, the data generated by the history and physical examination allowed for the study of disease in populations. Classifications of disease states followed and the fundamental science of epidemiology was established. The addition of laboratory results and diagnostic studies have allowed epidemiologists to further develop objectively measured categories of disease states and to study with greater precision the cause and effect relationships for these diseases. Advancements in treatment protocols for improved patient outcomes have thus evolved.

CLINICAL EPIDEMIOLOGY

According to Friedman (2004), there is a serious gap in understanding and communication between the scientifically-minded clinician and the epidemiologist. Epidemiologists and clinical scientists are primarily concerned with the study of relationships. Specifically, epidemiologists focus on the relationships between diseases and other human or environmental attributes by studying population groups. Clinicians focus their studies on the individual patient and they try to obtain complete and accurate information to provide the best possible diagnosis and treatment plan for that patient. Clinicians are very concerned about the individual patient's well-being; therefore he can tolerate few avoidable errors in this information. Based on their clinical training and knowledge, clinicians become accustomed to high standards in the pursuit of data and information, and spare no expense to acquire the information via laboratory, radiological, and diagnostic studies. With this in mind, many clinicians become intolerant of relatively low-quality data and information generated from the questionnaires, surveys, and death certificates used primarily in epidemiologic studies. The problem arises when clinicians perceive that information generated from large questionnaires and surveys are inferior because the clinician cannot physically examine and evaluate each patient included in the epidemiologic study. It is impossible to provide all the human and financial resources to provide for individual examination of each patient.

Epidemiological research, according to Friedman (2004), does not favor inferior data either. Epidemiological experience has been able to show that important relationships can be discerned, even if the data is of poor quality, because of the power of large quantities of data generated by studying large population groups. With some validity to the data and large enough numbers of study subjects to minimize sampling error, epidemiologists and other scientists may still be able to derive valuable information from poor-quality data. However, using poor data when better data is obtainable is not acceptable.

Epidemiologists are always aware of the limitations of the data used and the inaccuracies and biases which may affect the results of the study. Thus, data can be, and often are, so bad as to be unrevealing or even misleading, despite large numbers. Therefore, clinical epidemiology focuses on establishing the relationships between disease and human or environmental attributes. The individual examination of patients (when possible), along with using data generated by questionnaire and survey in large populations allows for valid, reliable, and accurate findings. These lead to improved outcomes with better diagnostic capabilities, and to treatment protocols that are the state of the art and thus can become the standard of care.

Healthcare Evaluation Design

INTRODUCTION TO HEALTHCARE EVALUATION DESIGN

The World Health Organization (WHO constitution, 1992) defines "health" as the:

> "State of complete physical, emotional, and social well-being, not merely the absence of disease or infirmity ... including intellectual, environmental, and spiritual health ... in an active process of becoming aware of and making choices toward a more successful existence"

Health can also be defined as the following:

- A condition or quality of the human organism which expresses adequate functioning under given genetic and environmental conditions. For example, an individual is healthy despite physical, psychological, and social challenges.
- An efficient performance of bodily functions taking place in the face of a wide range of changing environmental conditions. For example, an expression of adaptability.

Disease, on the other hand, is a pattern of responses to some form of insult or injury to the human body that results in disturbed psychological and biochemical function and/or structural, morphological alteration.

Understanding the difference between health and disease is important from the perspective of how one might measure outcomes within the healthcare delivery system. The healthcare delivery system must be defined so healthcare evaluation can be discussed. Healthcare delivery is any activity that has as its primary intention to improve and maintain individual and population health status and well-being through the continuum of care (e.g., preventive to acute to chronic to rehabilitative to palliative). In this discussion, the biopsychosocial approach (Engel, 1977, 1980) to healthcare delivery serves as the model for clinical services.

Healthcare delivery in the United States is provided by both a formal and informal system. Lay care is as important a determinate for improving and maintaining health status and well-being as professionally-delivered healthcare services. Determining whether the goals and objectives have been met allow for the evaluation of the success of the healthcare delivery system as a whole. This evaluation must be a critical assessment on as scientifically rigorous a basis as possible of the degree to which health services fulfill the stated goals and objectives providing valid, reliable data and information on quality and cost. The healthcare constituencies (see Table 8-1) who are paying for the services need to know whether they and those they are paying for to receive the healthcare services have received high quality, cost-efficient, easily accessible, customer-focused, and service-oriented healthcare delivery both at the point of care and within the delivery system as a whole.

Table 8-1   Health Services Research

Form of HSR	Focus of HSR
Disciplinary research	Theory
Basic Science research	Organisms
Clinical Science research	Individuals
Health Services research	System
Public Health research	Community

PURPOSE OF EVALUATING
HEALTHCARE·DELIVERY

The purpose of evaluating healthcare delivery is to provide treatments that work and not provide those that do not. There is a limit to the healthcare resources that can be made available for health care. The effort must be made to match the healthcare services provided to the needs of the population. Because health care is so expensive, it is necessary to choose those healthcare interventions that produce the greatest health gains at the lowest cost. Historical patterns of supply and demand have influenced the type and location of healthcare goods and services currently provided.

An assessment of quality or a judgment that aims to identify the "right thing to do" is the basic definition of evaluation. In making a judgment, a variety of modes of inquiry exist, extending from intuition to scientific analysis (see Figure 8-1). The cognitive continuum allows for both scientific analysis and intuition to contribute to the understanding of the process and structural complexity of the healthcare delivery system. Healthcare systems rely heavily on scientific analysis to find results that can be generalized to a larger context.

Often, traditional academic tertiary clinical research studies provide clinical information about less than one-tenth percent of the patients (White, 1961) who actually seek healthcare services. Important correlations related to the academic clinical research must be made at the point of care where the majority of patients in a community setting are accessing

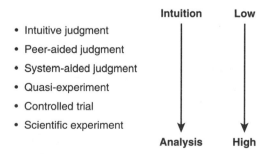

FIGURE 8-1 The Cognitive Continuum

healthcare delivery from their primary care physicians. Individual and population research studies on healthcare delivery must be applicable to the point of care in the community setting. Otherwise, the goals and objectives will not be met on any level and the healthcare delivery system cannot achieve success.

There are many levels today in which healthcare delivery can be studied (see Table 8-1). As previously discussed, the individual can be studied at the submolecular level all the way to the organ system level. The individual then becomes a part of the community and population and public health studies become the predominate forms of health services research.

Identifying the goals and objectives that need to be fulfilled in health services research requires that these goals and objectives are defined precisely. Goals are an expression of the fundamental tenants, directions, desired qualities, or market positions an organization seeks to achieve in healthcare delivery. Objectives are the actual health interventions that should be evaluated in their ability to fulfill specific statements of what an intervention is meant to do in the delivery of healthcare services. When evaluating a healthcare intervention, one must specify the objectives to be evaluated and these objectives must be measurable and as precise as possible. Goals are the endpoint of where the healthcare delivery system wants to be and objectives measure whether the goals have been achieved.

Outcomes are the results of any intervention occurring to patients and/or populations of patients in the healthcare delivery system. When evaluating healthcare services, one must choose and specify the outcomes to measure. Then, one can determine whether the objectives have been achieved by the healthcare delivery system. The exact nature of the outcomes specified depend on the nature of the intervention being studied in the health services research. For example, when evaluating a new day center for patients with mental illness, the outcomes measured might include the proportion of patients offered twice weekly attendance at the day center who subsequently require admission to a psychiatric hospital, the mean number of psychiatric admissions for patients attending the day center, and the reasons why patients who attend the day center require fewer psychiatric admissions. Simply knowing these facts is not sufficient to evaluate the service provided by the new mental health day center. Some specific standards are needed to assess healthcare outcomes.

FOUR DIMENSIONS OF HEALTHCARE EVALUATION

Jenkinson (1997) considers the following as specific standards that can be used to assess healthcare outcomes: effectiveness, efficiency, humanity, and equity. Effectiveness describes the benefits of health services measured by improvements in health in a real population. These improvements can be measured from a clinical performance perspective such as morbidity and mortality or from a quality of life perspective focusing on how an individual patient functions in daily living.

Efficiency compares the cost of an intervention to the benefits obtained by the individual or population being studied. Ideally the benefits should be measured in terms of the degree of health gained, again based on a clinical perspective or a quality of life measure. This dimension is difficult to measure because of the paucity of models available to study efficiency.

Humanity is described as having a quality of being humane, sharing emotionally with individual patients as they interact with clinicians in the healthcare delivery system. Humanity also describes the social, psychological, and ethical acceptability of the treatment that people receive from healthcare interventions. Unfortunately, inhumanity may be more easily recognized during patient care (e.g., forced restraints of patients) than humane treatment. Humanity as a dimension of healthcare evaluation is measured from the individual or population perspective as satisfaction with the delivery of services. The actual interpersonal relationships can be evaluated from many perspectives within the healthcare delivery system including clinicians, support staff, facilities, and overall operational characteristics that the individual patient interacts with during his/her care encounter.

The final dimension, equity, describes the fair distribution of both the benefits and the burdens of health services among individuals and populations being studied. This dimension evaluates the access to both healthcare services and to public health measures that evaluate ethical and social issues of healthcare services.

When a new healthcare intervention is introduced into healthcare delivery as a new service, it should be evaluated based on these four dimensions. When comparing alternative established interventions, it may be sufficient to evaluate only those dimensions that are likely to differ between the interventions. However, it is always necessary to decide and state which dimensions should be evaluated so that the study parameters resulting from the study can be properly framed and discussed. Whether an intervention is appropriate for a population or individual is related to the healthcare evaluation dimensions. If an intervention is not appropriate for a given individual, it will either be because this intervention is less effective or efficient than an alternative, or because it is simply not humane or equitable (perhaps for sociocultural reasons).

The point of view from which healthcare delivery is studied and the dimensions chosen to evaluate from an outcomes perspective depend on the goals and objectives established at the outset of the study. The different perspectives of the health constituencies and the different purposes for the determination of the outcomes are determined by society or institutional beliefs, desires, and agendas. This is what determines the design and development of the studies.

HEALTHCARE EVALUATION DESIGN AND DEVELOPMENT

The healthcare evaluation process seeks to measure how a change in the way that care is provided affects the health and well-being of individuals or populations. This process works by comparing one form of health care with another or with no care at all. The different forms of health care provided to individuals or populations are compared in terms of the four dimensions of healthcare evaluation previously discussed: effectiveness, efficiency, humanity, and equity. The evaluation design process begins by describing the goals and objectives of the evaluation. The process needs to be precise, contain a description of the intervention(s) that will be evaluated, and contain a description of the population who will receive the intervention(s).

The healthcare evaluation dimensions to be evaluated must be chosen; these dimensions depend on the nature of the healthcare intervention(s) and the perspective from which the evaluation will be undertaken. Outcomes planning and management requires that the chosen dimensions must be determined at the outset of the study to provide clarity and value at the conclusion of the study. The study design must be developed so that it can evaluate the chosen dimensions by which appropriate data sources can be identified, queried, analyzed, and reported at the conclusion of the study.

There are a wide range of methods for studying healthcare delivery services and systems. One method is qualitative in nature. This method answers the question "what?" The other method is quantitative and answers the question, "how often?" Data collection and analysis can be based on whether an individual or a population is chosen to be the subject of the evaluation. Some methods are chosen because they are better suited to the healthcare evaluation dimension studied.

All methods seek to eliminate bias, errors, and confounding. Bias indicates systematic error within the study. Bias occurs when data relating to one group of patients are treated differently from the data relating to the other groups of patients. As a result, any difference in measured outcomes between the groups may be due to bias. Confounding arises when there is a factor that is associated with both the intervention (new or standard treatment) and the outcome, but is not part of the way that the intervention causes the outcome. There will be a more thorough discussion on bias and confounding when experimental healthcare evaluations are discussed in detail later in this chapter.

To better understand study design and development, let us suppose that a healthcare evaluation study seeks to evaluate a new technology in healthcare delivery. The criteria that a new healthcare technology must satisfy before it should be introduced into use for patient care should be to improve the health outcomes that actually matter to patients, produce greater amount of benefit than harm, produce health benefits that are worth the cost incurred to introduce the new technology, and deserve priority over other technologies competing for the same resources.

To describe how well the study measures the effects of the new healthcare technology, the internal validity of the study must be established. Internal validity also describes how well the study measures "efficacy"; it relates the population taking part in the study to the circumstances of care that they will receive. On the other hand, external validity describes how well the effects of this new healthcare technology can be expected to apply to patients outside of the study environment. If the study population is highly selective it may not represent those who will actually need the healthcare technology in the wider community. Therefore, the same degree of effectiveness as measured in the current study is unlikely.

Fundamental to determining the internal and external validity of any study, or for that matter, eliminating bias, errors, and confounding begins at the outset of the research. Research methodology is a particular strategy for answering a proposed research question. This strategy includes formulating a research question, providing a general design of the study, surveying the population to be studied, designing an experiment to answer the research question, and developing tools to gather data including questionnaires and interviewing participants in the study.

In formulating the research question, the study objective can be established by searching for other relevant research, carrying out an original research project, or commissioning a larger project from an experienced researcher in a related area of interest. The applied medical sciences are often extensions of the classical social sciences such as sociology, psychology, and anthropology. Both disciplines study aspects of human behavior. Research in this arena is relevant when a problem relates to some aspect of human behavior or attitude, individually or with a population.

Effectiveness, efficiency, and acceptability of healthcare systems are influenced by human behavior and attitude at many levels. Social science methodologies are often relevant and applicable to designing research studies in the applied medical sciences. Research questions in applied medical science research can be either qualitative or quantitative in nature. Qualitative research questions explore the meaning of events and phenomena. Quantitative research questions address measurement.

In answering the research question, strict adherence to science and scientific methodology has been accepted by many to exist in the applied medical sciences. Work by Engel (1977, 1980) established that scientific methodology can result in answers to subjective questions in clinical medicine. Scientific methodology requires detailed observation and accurate measurement of phenomena that can be detected with the physical sciences or extensions of these senses. Applied to the social sciences, scientific methodology applies a range of approaches and methods resulting in subjective findings that can be influenced by the attitude of the researcher.

In a controlled experiment, regardless of if it is objective or subjective in nature, the researcher is aware of all conditions, and controls the conditions. For example, the experimental group is exposed to the intervention and the control group is not. Formulating a good hypothesis in terms that allow predictions, which can be tested either by observation or experimentation, to be made is critical for the success of the healthcare evaluation research study.

POSITIVISM VERSUS RELATIVISM

There have been two significant philosophies established and debated as to which is most appropriate to study applied medical phenomena such as healthcare delivery of services. These philosophies are *positivism* and *relativism*. Positivism (Marks et al., 2000) is defined as the philosophy that holds that there are laws governing behavior in the natural world, and that the proper object of science is to discover them. To accomplish this discovery, scientists must study observable phenomena, which can be objectively measured and then reported. This view has had a significant influence on many social science methods over many years of social science research. In summary, positivism is the study of observable facets of human behavior, which can be measured, and attempting to derive general laws about behavior from their observations.

An example of positivism can best be described by the work of sociologist Emil Durkheim, a nineteenth century French classical theorist (Cockerham, 2004). Durkheim studied the records of suicide rates across Europe. He discovered that different societies had different propensities to suicide based upon factors such as religion, socioeconomic status, marital status, etc. He developed a positivist theory that linked the rate of suicide (observable facts) to the lack of social integration in a society (a general law from the data measured, recorded, and analyzed).

Relativism (Marks et al., 2000), on the other hand, follows the philosophy that assumes no one, stable reality that pre-exists for scientists to discover. In fact, realities, and our knowledge of that reality, are socially constructed—they are a product of the particular social, political, and historical circumstances. Relativists do not believe that observable facts are objective facts that reflect an underlying reality about the observable fact or the existence of disease in an individual. For example, symptoms of disease are classified in different ways in different countries based upon culture, socioeconomic status, educational level, etc.

In summary, positivists believe that there is a stable reality which research should strive to represent in the applied medical sciences. Contrarily, relativists believe that reality is constructed differently, and depends on who is looking at it and from where.

QUALITATIVE AND QUANTITATIVE RESEARCH METHODOLOGY

Regardless of whether one is a positivist or a relativist, research methodology in healthcare evaluation remains either qualitative or quantitative in nature. Qualitative research methods are characterized as those which aim to explore meaning and traditionally produce non-numerical data. Data collection techniques using qualitative research methodology include participant observation, in-depth interviewing, focus groups, and analyzing textual or pictorial data.

What makes a research design qualitative is the aim of the study and how the data produced are analyzed, not the data collection strategy itself. The common aim in all qualitative research is informing policy makers about the experiences and attitudes of the patients, the community, or healthcare deliverers. According to medical sociologists Fitzpatrick and Boulton (1994):

> Qualitative research depends upon not numerical but conceptual analysis and presentation. It is used where it is important to understand the meaning and interpretation of human social arrangements such as hospitals, clinics, forms of management, or decision making. Qualitative methods are intended to convey to policy makers the experiences of individuals, groups, and organizations that may be affected by policies.

Quantitative research methodology, on the other hand, has a number of techniques for quantifying aspects of social life. Quantitative research methodology uses standardized and scheduled questionnaires and employs the statistical manipulation of numerical analysis as the main method of analysis. The main advantages of using quantitative research methodology over qualitative research methodology are the ability to discern patterns over time (e.g., illness, disease), to give the impression of certainty, and to provide useful illustration of trends. The disadvantages of quantitative research are the ways in which statistical tables or other sources of numerical data have been constructed over time, that figures are not themselves value-free, that figures raise questions of interpretation, and that conclusions drawn from this type of data are as subjective as those drawn from qualitative source material.

EXPERIMENTAL HEALTHCARE EVALUATIONS

According to Jekel et al. (1996), science is based on the following principles: previous experience serves as the basis for developing hypotheses, hypotheses serve as the basis for developing predictions, and predictions must be subjected to experimental or observational testing. Experimental healthcare evaluation primarily uses only two out of the four healthcare dimensions described by Jenkinson (1997)—effectiveness and efficacy.

To review, effectiveness describes the benefits of health services measured by improvements in health in a real population. These improvements can be measured from a clinical performance perspective, such as morbidity and mortality or from a quality of life perspective that focuses on individual patient's functionality in daily living. Efficiency compares the cost of an intervention to the benefits obtained by the individual or population being studied. Ideally the benefits should be measured in terms of the degree of health gained, again either from a clinical perspective or from a quality of life measure. This dimension is difficult to measure because of the paucity of models available to study efficiency. The importance of using either dimension relates to whether a statistical association exists between an outcome and the intervention being studied. Without demonstrating a statistical association, the strength of reporting on either effectiveness or efficacy of an intervention in healthcare delivery is significantly diminished.

To show that a valid statistical association exists, the outcome must be linked to the intervention (i.e., they are "associated" with one another). The association is not simply due to chance and the P-value (as it was previously defined) represents a true deviation from what was to be expected (the hypothesis). The association is not due to bias or confounding; the integrity of internal validity can be established and verified.

The assessment of internal validity for an experimental healthcare evaluation's association between an outcome and an intervention relies upon establishing whether bias and confounding have affected the findings in the study. Bias and confounding can produce the appearance of an association that does not exist and can prevent the appearance of an association that really does exist. Bias can be described as a "systematic error" in the design of the experimental healthcare evaluation and arises when the groups of patients experiencing different treatments differ in ways that are not due simply to chance. There are four types of bias including selection bias, observation bias, interviewer bias, and responder bias.

Selection bias arises if the enrollment of patients into a study group is influenced by a particular patient characteristic. For example, very ill patients were selected to receive the new experimental treatment on the grounds that they were unlikely to benefit from the standard (relatively ineffective) treatment. Observation bias can be described as an error in measurement that is introduced by the investigator or observer of the study. For example, patients receiving the new treatment were reviewed in clinic more often than those who received the standard treatment. Interviewer bias, a form of observational bias, occurs when an interviewer treats patients from different study groups in different manners. For example, an interviewer knows that the new treatment given to the study's patients is likely to cause abdominal pain. The interviewer also knows which patients received the new treatment and which patients did not receive the new treatment. It is then possible that the interviewer might ask those who received the new treatment more searching questions about abdominal pain and bias the results of the intervention and therefore the outcomes. Finally, responder bias, also a form of observational bias, occurs when the patients are more likely to report certain information according to the study group they have been allocated into, either the new intervention group or the control group. Confounding arises when there is a factor that is associated with both the intervention (new or standard treatment) and the outcome, but is not part of the way that the intervention causes the outcome.

How can bias be avoided in an experimental healthcare evaluation? First, selection bias can be avoided by randomly allocating patients into the appropriate study groups. However, it is important to ensure that each study group is similar for case-mix characteristics (e.g., age, gender, severity of illness). Observation bias can be avoided by providing the same follow-up to each study group of patients. For example, there should be the same clinic appointments and clinical protocol for all subjects in all study groups. Interviewer bias can be avoided by actually "blinding the interviewer." Here, the interviewer or observer recording information on the study groups does not know which treatment was received by which patient. This is much easier to do with medical interventions compared to surgical interventions because of the scar on the skin from the intervention. Finally, responder bias can be avoided by "blinding the responder." In this manner, the patients are unaware of which treatment they are receiving as part of the study group.

To avoid confounding, one should list all known or likely confounding variables (i.e., age, gender) at the beginning of the study and allocate patients to each study group in a way that these variables are equally represented in each group (e.g., same number of men and women in each study group).

Another important facet of any experimental healthcare evaluation relates to whether the data and information gathered from the research study can be applied to other patients outside of the study. After all, this is the motivating factor for undertaking clinical research. A healthcare evaluation research study can only measure the association between health interventions and outcomes in those patients who actually take part in the study itself. To be of relevance to the wider population, the study's results must be applicable to other patients with similar illnesses. The intervention of the study should produce the same degree of effectiveness and efficacy when used in the community-at-large at the point of care. External validity or generalizability is increased when the patients who take part in the study represent patients with the same condition in the general population.

Causality is another important issue that must be considered when performing healthcare evaluations. It is important to look for a cause-and-effect relationship between an intervention and the outcome. In other words, the research study should be able to demonstrate that the intervention (exposure) causes the effect. This requires a valid statistical association between the intervention and the outcome.

There are well-established criteria that allow for the cause and effect relationship between an intervention and outcome to be established. First, the strength of association between the intervention and outcome is established. If the intervention greatly increases the chance of the outcome the association is more likely to be causal. For example, smoking greatly increases the risk of lung cancer. Second, biological credibility or plausibility must be established. It is easier to believe that an intervention causes an outcome if evidence already exists to show how this might occur. Third, there must be consistent evidence that the cause-and-effect relationship is established by other research studies. If multiple studies agree on causality, the relationship between intervention and outcome is more evident. Fourth, the time sequence at which the cause and effect is established provides evidence that the relationship exists. The intervention (cause) pre-dates the outcome (effect). Finally, there is a dose-response relationship that enables the cause and effect to be established. If an increase in the amount of the intervention is associated with an increase in the chance of experiencing the outcome, a causal relationship is suggested. For example, the chance of survival increases as the dose of a drug increases.

RANDOMIZED CONTROL TRIAL— THE GOLD STANDARD OF EXPERIMENTAL EVALUATIONS IN HEALTH CARE

The randomized control trial (RCT) is the gold standard for performing all experimental healthcare evaluations. The RCT is an experimental study where each patient is allocated to a treatment group (or treatment arm) of a research study that investigates the relationship between an intervention (cause) and its outcomes (effect). This allocation of patients occurs so that neither the investigator nor the patient can predict the treatment that will be received. The patients are treated using strict clinical protocols, and followed to determine the outcomes occurring in each treatment group of the research study. This randomization helps to prevent selection bias and is intended to distribute both known and unknown confounding variables equally between treatment and control groups participating in the research study.

There are two main types of RCTs—explanatory RCTs and pragmatic RCTs. The explanatory RCTs measure efficacy and require that patients entering the study be as similar as possible. The results of an explanatory RCT may not be generalizable to the population-at-large. The pragmatic RCTs measure effectiveness and aim to recruit a sample of patients who represent the wider patient population and typical health services.

The advantages of performing RCTs are many. All investigators pay explicit attention to potential sources of error. This is one of the reasons for the RCTs high standing as a scientifically rigorous evaluation method. RCTs generally have high internal validity. Because it is an experiment, patient selection and the conditions of the treatment can be precisely controlled.

With its ability to reduce bias and to distribute confounding variables equally, the RCT can provide a precise estimate of a treatment's effects under experimental conditions. Carefully following the established clinical research protocol, RCTs often have a reduction of bias built into the design and development of the research study. Random allocation reduces selection bias provided that the allocation is followed properly. Observation bias is reduced by blinding. In a single blinded study, the patient does not know the treatment allocation group for which he/she is assigned. In a double blinded study, neither the patient nor investigator know to which group the patient has been assigned. It is important to note, however, that the RCTs cannot remove errors associated with recall and response bias, but the clinical research protocol ensures equal chances of it occurring in either treatment arm.

A final advantage for RCTs as an experimental research study is that they allow for the reduction of confounding. Some types of studies control for confounding variables in their design by assigning an equal number of age and gender to each treatment arm of the study. Only RCTs can control for unknown confounders. The experimental research study must be large enough for chance to balance unknown confounding variables evenly between the study arms.

The disadvantages of RCTs are also abundant. The timing of the trial must be considered. There is a relatively short time period after the introduction of a new therapy during which an RCT can be performed because of a low level of clinical expertise by investigators with a new therapy, the randomization may be unethical in that it may expose patients to an untested therapy, and the results at this stage may be poor reflecting the low level of clinician/investigator expertise. A long time-scale is required to complete the study. For example, all prospective studies suffer if there is a need for prolonged follow-up with the patients participating in the study because tracing participants becomes difficult over time.

The actual cost of the study can be a significant disadvantage. The RCT can be very expensive to design, develop, and conduct because it can cause significant changes to working practices. Personnel changes and overtime must occur cover for personnel involved in conducting the study. In addition, the cost for purchasing new equipment and for training persons to use this equipment can be significant in initiating an experimental study.

With many ethical changes, human rights, and informed consent requirements added to all health intervention studies within the past several years, it is necessary to explain the nature and purpose of any experimental trial to potential subjects in full detail outlining potential risks and benefits so that full disclosure can be guaranteed to all the potential participants. Again, this requires money to pay for adequate staffing of the study to ensure its proper attention to clinical protocol.

The issue of generalizability may be affected. Subjects enrolled in a RCT study should accurately represent the total population from which they were drawn. In other words, these are the people who should benefit from the new treatment if it shown to be beneficial. However, RCTs may suffer from a lack of external validity due to too strict inclusion criteria, having a large proportion of patients refuse randomization, and having undetected differences between those participants who accept randomization and those that do not.

Patient and clinician preferences can result in a disadvantage for the RCTs. Some therapies have as a major component of their beneficial effect the clinician's or patient's belief that the person will get well. Randomization and blinding can effectively remove this element, thereby enhancing the effectiveness of the intervention.

Compliance and crossover issues can have an adverse impact on the results of the RCT. Failure to comply with clinical protocol that appropriately allocates treatment can lead to an under- or overestimate of effectiveness as it applies to the population-at-large. Crossover in an experimental research study occurs when, based on clinical protocol, patients are changing treatment arms during the study. As a result of crossover, dilution within the study population can occur, resulting in patients of one study arm receiving less of their allocated treatment. In addition, contamination can occur during crossover; patients therefore receive an alternative study treatment and the potential relationship between the intervention and the outcome is affected.

The design and development of RCTs requires attention to the following details: selection of subjects, sample size, trial design, and ethical issues. The selection of subjects for a RCT is the process by which a sample of patients for the study is identified. The better the patients selected for the RCT represent the patient population, the more generalizable the RCT will be. The steps required for selecting patients include the following:

1. Defining the RCT population or identifying the type of patient to recruit and where to recruit them (i.e., an outpatient clinic).
2. Developing inclusion criteria or features that all potential RCT subjects must have to be eligible to participate in the RCT.

3. Developing exclusion criteria or features that all potential RCT subjects must not have to be eligible to participate in the RCT.
4. Designing a recruitment process to identify eligible potential RCT participants and invite them to participate in the trial.

The sample size of the RCT participants is the number of patients who need to be recruited to each treatment arm of the RCT. There is a need to study the "right number" of patients for many reasons including limited resources, ethical considerations, and removing chance as the reason for the observed difference in outcomes (i.e., achieving the desired level of statistical significance). In order to select the right number of subjects for the RCT, the expected difference in outcomes between the treatment arms that would be considered to be clinically or socially significant must be decided. For example, if an RCT expects a large difference in outcome between treatment arms of the study, then a smaller sample size of participants is needed. Additionally to select the right number of subjects for the RCT, a decision must be made on the degree of statistical significance that eliminate the factor of chance. The statistical significance is usually set at a five percent level where a p-value of .05 means that there is a five percent (or 1 in 20 chance) probability that the results of the RCT or the outcomes could be due to chance alone.

The power of the study measures the chance of detecting a difference between the treatment arms of the RCT. For example, how likely is the RCT to detect a significant difference in outcomes? The larger the samples size of participants in the RCT, the higher the power of the RCT and vice versa.

From an ethical perspective, the RCTs performed today must follow the principles that are contained in the 1964 Declaration of Helsinki. It is the mission of the clinician to safeguard the health of the human participants. His or her knowledge and conscience are dedicated to the fulfillment of this mission. The World Medical Association's Declaration of Geneva (1996) binds the physician with the words, "The health of my patient will be my first consideration," and the International Code of Medical Ethics declares that, "A physician shall act only in the patient's interest when providing medical care which might have the effect of weakening the physical and mental condition of the patient."

The purpose of biomedical research involving human subjects must be to improve diagnostic, therapeutic, and prophylactic procedures and the understanding of the etiology and pathogenesis of disease. In current medical practice most diagnostic, therapeutic, or prophylactic procedures involve hazards. This applies especially to biomedical research. Medical progress is based on research which ultimately must rest in part on experimentation involving human subjects.

A fundamental distinction must be made between medical research in which the aim is essentially diagnostic or therapeutic for a patient and medical research in which the aim is purely scientific without implying direct diagnostic or therapeutic value to the person subjected to the research. Special caution must be exercised in the conduct of research which may affect the environment and the welfare of animals used for research must be respected. Because it is essential that the results of laboratory experiments be applied to human beings to further scientific knowledge and to help suffering humanity, the World Medical Association (1996) has prepared the following recommendations as a guide to every physician in biomedical research involving human subjects. They should be kept under review in the future. It must be stressed that the standards as drafted are only a guide for physicians all over the world. Physicians are not relieved from criminal, civil, and ethical responsibilities under the law of their own countries.

I. Basic principles of biomedical research

1. Biomedical research involving human subjects must conform to generally accept scientific principles and should be based on adequately performed laboratory and animal experimentation and on a thorough knowledge of the scientific literature.

2. The design and performance of each experimental procedure involving human subjects should be clearly formulated in an experimental protocol which should be transmitted to a specially appointed independent committee for consideration, comment, and guidance.

3. Biomedical research involving human subjects should be conducted only by scientifically qualified persons and under the supervision of a clinically competent medical person. The responsibility for the human subject must always rest with a medically qualified person and never rest on the subject of the research, even though the subject has given his or her consent.

4. Biomedical research involving human subjects cannot legitimately be carried out unless the importance of the objective is in proportion to the inherent risk to the subject.

5. Every biomedical research project involving human subjects should be preceded by careful assessment of predictable risks in comparison with foreseeable benefits to the subject or to others. Concern for the interests of the subject must always prevail over the interests of science and society.

6. The right of the research subject to safeguard his or her integrity must always be respected. Every precaution should be taken to respect the privacy of the subject and to minimize the impact of the study on the subject's physical and mental integrity and on the personality of the subject.

7. Physicians should abstain from engaging in research projects involving human subjects unless they are satisfied that the hazards involved are believed to be predictable. Physicians should cease any investigation if the hazards are found to outweigh the potential benefits.

8. In publication of the results of his or her research, the physician is obliged to preserve the accuracy of the results. Reports of experimentation not in accordance with the principles laid down in this Declaration should not be accepted for publication.

9. In any research on human beings, each potential subject must be adequately informed of the aims, methods, anticipated benefits, and potential hazards of the study and the discomfort it may entail. He or she should be informed that he or she is at liberty to abstain from participation in the study and that he or she is free to withdraw visor her consent to participation at any time. The physician should then obtain the subject's freely given informed consent, preferably in writing.

10. When obtaining informed consent for the research project the physician should be particularly cautious if the subject is in dependent relationship to him or her or may consent under duress. In that case the informed consent should be obtained by a physician who isn't engaged in

the investigation and who is completely independent of this official relationship.

11. In case of legal incompetence, informed consent should be obtained from the legal guardian in accordance with national legislation. Where physical or mental incapacity makes it impossible to obtain informed consent, or when the subject is a minor, permission from the responsible relative replaces that of the subject in accordance with national legislation. Whenever the minor child is in fact able to give consent, the minor's consent must be obtained in addition to the consent of the minor's legal guardian.

12. The research protocol should always contain a statement of the ethical considerations involved and should indicate that the principles enunciated in the present declaration are complied with.

II. Medical research combined with professional care or clinical research

1. In the treatment of the sick person, the physician must be free to use a new diagnostic and therapeutic measure, if in his or her judgment it offers hope of saving life, re-establishing health or alleviating suffering.

2. The potential benefits, hazards and discomfort of a new method should be weighed against the advantages of the best current diagnostic and therapeutic methods.

3. In any medical study, every patient—including those of a control group, if any—should be assured of the best proven diagnostic and therapeutic method.

4. The refusal of the patient to participate in a study must never interfere with the physician–patient relationship.

5. If the physician considers it essential not to obtain informed consent, the specific reasons for this proposal should be stated in the experimental protocol for transmission to the independent committee.

6. The physician can combine medical research with professional care, the objective being the acquisition of new medical knowledge, only to the extent that medical research is justified by its potential diagnostic or therapeutic value for the patient.

III. Non-therapeutic biomedical research involving human subjects or non-clinical biomedical research

1. In the purely scientific application of medical research carried out on a human being, it is the duty of the physician to remain the protector of the life and health of that person on whom biomedical research is being carried out.

2. The subjects should be volunteers—either healthy persons or patients for whom the experimental design is not related to the patient's illness.

3. The investigator or the investigating team should discontinue the research if in his/her or their judgment it may, if continued, be harmful to the individual.

4. In research on man, the interest of science and society should never take precedence over considerations related to the well-being of the subject.

OBSERVATIONAL HEALTHCARE EVALUATIONS

Observational healthcare evaluations examine the effects of health care without influencing the care that is provided or the patients who receive it. These evaluations do not require any change in the way healthcare services are delivered at the point of care. Observational healthcare evaluations can be either prospective or retrospective in nature. In a prospective evaluation, patients and interventions are identified and subsequently followed to determine the outcomes. In contrast, the retrospective evaluation studies patients who have already received their treatment and experienced outcomes as a result of the treatment.

Observational healthcare evaluations take the place of RCTs in situations where RCTs are unnecessary, inappropriate, impossible, or inadequate. An unnecessary situation not suitable for a RCT is where there is a very dramatic large benefit to the population-at-large. Inappropriate situations not suitable for a RCT include measuring rare adverse outcomes, detecting the reduction of rare harmful events, detecting outcomes in the far future, and determining if the benefits of the intervention depend partly on the active participation of the patient. Impossible situations not suitable for a RCT include clinicians who refuse to participate in the study, ethical objections by participants or investigators, political obstacles, legal obstacles, contamination of the study groups, and interventional tasks that are too large. Finally, inadequate situations not suitable for a RCT include when the participating professionals, the patients, and/or the treatment are atypical with respects to the community-at-large.

Other issues limit RCTs from being used in observational studies. First, RCTs ignore the context of the participants' attitudes and beliefs. Second, RCTs may become necessary after an observational study reveals a level of uncertainty about an intervention. Finally, RCTs cannot investigate all interventions such as those that study managerial reorganization and different mechanisms of financing health care.

There are three main types of observational studies to discuss: cohort studies, case-control studies, and ecological studies. The cohort study observes patients exposed to a risk factor and subsequently follows up to determine whether this exposure was associated with particular adverse outcomes. Patients' exposures may be due to different treatments rather than risk factors, and the outcomes are measured in terms of health gain or loss, functionality, or quality of life. Cohorts can be organized into different groups of patients receiving alternative interventions and they can be analyzed in a prospective versus retrospective outcomes analysis. In a prospective cohort study, one may compare the complication rates of giving birth at home with those of giving birth in a hospital. Questions of relevance to in determining what to study prospectively may include:

- What interventions to compare?
- What are the inclusion and exclusion criteria?
- How and when to collect data?
- How to control for confounders?
- How to analyze the data?

Enlisting the support of relevant healthcare workers and facilities is critical to the success of the study. Consecutive patients must be invited to participate. Confounding factors such as age and the status of the pregnancy (e.g., uncomplicated vs. complicated) along with other detailed information must be determined for all participants. Appropriate health outcomes to be collected are determined prior to the study and analysis comparing the outcomes of the two cohorts (after adjusting for confounding variables) can begin as data is collected.

Contrarily, retrospective studies identify groups of patients who have experienced the interventions in the past. This defined period of time actually defines the cohorts. Using the same example, one can look back and compare the complication rates of pregnant women who gave birth at home with those who gave birth in a hospital. Retrospective cohort studies also require the collection of all available information on known confounders such as age and severity of the pregnancy, and if it was uncomplicated or complicated. Immediate and long-term health outcomes can be determined and data can be collected for analysis comparing the two cohorts (after adjusting for confounding variables) in much the same way as a prospective cohort study.

Observational healthcare evaluations using the cohort model must carefully consider ethical issues presented in any other research study. Even though an observational study does not require any changes in the healthcare services that patients receive, it does involve collecting data about patients. Therefore administering questionnaires and interviewing patients must be considered an integral part of the study protocol. Ethical goals of the cohort study include ensuring that patients are treated fairly and without prejudice to their care, that studies are performed only if they seek to provide answers to important clinical problems, and that there is no unnecessary inconvenience to patients.

The main threats to the validity of a cohort study are confounding and bias. Cohort studies cannot use randomization to evenly distribute unknown confounding variables. In addition, cohort studies cannot blind patients or staff to the treatment allocations. However, the investigators can be blinded when evaluating health outcomes. Then the analysis of the data can be improved for a more meaningful clinical application to the community-at-large.

Losing participants to follow up can adversely impact the analysis of outcomes data in a cohort study. To mitigate this potential problem, investigators must make every effort to obtain outcome data from all participants in the study, especially if there is no difference between the follow-up of each cohort. Simple and consistent procedures for follow-up must be developed and implemented in the study protocol.

Selection, observation, interviewer, and recall bias can also impact the analysis of a cohort study; however the impact of bias can be reduced to enhance the validity of the cohort study. For example, selection bias can be mitigated by measuring all known confounders and by taking any differences between the treatment groups into account in the analysis of the outcomes data. Observation and interviewer bias can be mitigated by making the data collection procedure as precise and consistent as possible, by training investigators to ensure they ask all participants the same questions in exactly the same way, by having patients examined by a blinded investigator, and by reviewing the study records during the analysis phase of the study. Recall bias is very difficult to control. Often, major events are more likely to be recalled than minor events and recent events are more likely to be recalled than past events.

Case-control studies are the second type of observational healthcare evaluations. Patients are defined as cases or controls on the basis of the outcome of their clinical care. Patients are then investigated to determine which interventions they have received. The study aims to determine whether a statistical association exists between the outcome and the intervention. Case-control studies are largely confined to the evaluation of age-related preventive healthcare interventions. More specifically, a case can be defined as an individual manifesting a particular health outcome. A control can be defined as an individual who does not manifest a particular health outcome. Individuals selected as controls should be similar to the individuals selected as cases *except* for the risk factors that are being investigated in the study.

Case-control studies are good for investigating rare outcomes and several different risk factors in the same study. It is only possible to consider one outcome in a case-control study. It is important to note that it is the outcome that defines whether a patient is a case or a control. To illustrate how this type of observational study works, let us look at a hypothetical example. It has been suggested that vitamin E may reduce the incidence of certain forms of cancer. One could test this suggestion by randomizing individuals to take vitamin E capsules or not. One could set up a prospective cohort study to compare individuals who happen to be taking vitamin E with others who are not. One would have to wait years to discover the effects of vitamin E on cancer incidence. Before designing a case-control study, some basic questions must be answered:

- How would you define:
  - The cases and controls for this study?
  - The exposure?
- What would you expect to find if vitamin E really did provide protection from these forms of cancer?

To begin, the "cases" are people with a diagnosis of one of the relevant forms of cancer, and the "controls" are people without such cancers. Next, one must determine the exposure of cases and controls to the treatment or risk factor of interest (the exposure would be vitamin E). Then, the investigator determines the proportion of cases and the proportion of controls that had diets containing high concentrations of vitamin E or who took vitamin E supplements. If vitamin E is really protective against cancer, what would you expect to see in the cases versus the controls? One would expect the cases to show a lower consumption of vitamin E than the controls.

There are many advantages to using the case-control observational healthcare evaluation. First, it is effective when studying rare adverse outcomes. As the cases are defined by their having experienced the outcome of interest, it is possible to investigate adverse outcomes that are rare; for example deaths following straightforward surgery for benign conditions, or mental impairment following whooping cough vaccination. The speed at which a case-control study can be performed and the lower cost to perform the study is another great advantage. Because case-control study is a retrospective study, the health outcome has already occurred and there is no need to wait for patients to experience it. Therefore this study is easy and inexpensive. Third, ethical issues with case-control studies are easier to define and address. Ethical issues in case-control studies do not involve any change to the treatment patients receive. In fact, because case-control studies are retrospective, the study does not influence the health outcomes at all.

The disadvantages of case-control studies center on bias and causal uncertainty. Case-control studies are susceptible to selection bias. Therefore, investigators must choose controls. In addition, data collection may be subject to recall bias because this type of study is retrospective by design. Prospective studies can usually determine that healthcare interventions occur before outcomes. This is not the case with case-control studies. This type of observational study requires that the outcome is identified first. If the outcome is a disease with a long latent period, the disease may have pre-dated the healthcare intervention, resulting in an adverse result on the data collection and interpretation.

The threats to validity using case-control studies are the same compared to cohort studies—bias and confounding. Techniques to reduce the effect of confounding are restriction and matching of the study participants. Restriction can be used to avoid the effects of a confounding variable by ensuring that patients in each study group (i.e., cases and controls) are affected in the same way by this confounder. For example, if smoking is the confounding variable, then the study could be restricted to include only smokers or non-smokers. Matching can be used as each case is matched with a particular control with regard to the presence of a confounding variable. For example, each case who smokes would be matched with a control who smokes a similar amount and each non-smoking case would be matched with a non-smoking control.

The most important source of bias in the design of case-control studies is selection bias. Ideally, controls and cases should be identical in every way except the outcome of interest and the exposure that causes this outcome. Whether an individual is selected as a case or control may be based on if this individual was exposed to the risk factor of interest. Selecting controls is one of the most important aspects of design when using this type of observational evaluation.

The final observational healthcare evaluation to discuss here is the ecological study. An ecological study studies the population or group rather than the individual. Data representing a particular group in this type of study do not give any indication of how individuals vary within the group, or indicate if any variation is similar in different groups. Ecological studies are designed to rely on data from healthcare delivery services compared with those on outcomes in a population. There is no attempt made to identify individuals receiving healthcare services or to relate the intervention to health outcomes for individuals. For example, international differences in infant mortality, staffing levels of health centers and vaccination rates, and equity of access to care between regions are just a few ways in which the ecological observational evaluation could be used.

Advantages to using ecological studies include the ability to produce results for little cost by taking advantage of routine data sources and exploiting the natural variations between groups or between different time periods (e.g., the introduction of a new intervention). The only feasible way of evaluating the effects of healthcare programs where data on individuals' outcomes are not available is the ecological observational evaluation. Other advantages include the ability to provide the appropriate strategy for assessing changes in legislation or health poli-cies, such as health promotion campaigns, that are aimed at groups and for generating hypotheses to be investigated at the individual level. This would then result in the use of a cohort or case-control study to follow up on the hypothesis.

The disadvantages to using an ecological observational study center on the "ecological fallacy," which is also considered ecological bias. The eco-logical fallacy can be defined as whether the effects measured on groups can be applicable at the individual level. For example, if a community receives a new, easily accessible health center, will the health of the people using the health center improve? The health improvement may not actu-ally occur in the people who attend the new health center. Therefore, the improvement may be falsely attributed to the new facility.

The two major types of ecological designs are the time-series and the multiple group analysis. The time-series design looks at group-level varia-tions over a time in a defined population. Secular trends of disease rele-vant in a healthcare evaluation are examined. This is the simplest design because the health outcome is measured at one time before and at one time after the new intervention has been introduced (e.g., perinatal mor-tality and the introduction of a new mother-child healthcare program). The multiple group analysis relies on determining the rate of disease in a population. This rate is measured in a number of different groups or pop-ulations during the same time period and used to identify spatial patterns of disease (e.g., determining the prevalence of childhood cancer near a nuclear power plant).

Ecological observational studies can also have problems with their study design and development. Examples of these problems include the following:

- When trying to identify an attribution between health outcomes and an intervention
- When studying concurrent interventions that change the health outcome
- When the intervention to be evaluated is diffuse and phased in over a long period of time
- When the healthcare intervention to be evaluated has a long latent period, long period of time between the intervention and effect (e.g., changes in tobacco laws and the decline in lung cancer mortality)

CONCLUSION

Measuring healthcare outcomes within the healthcare delivery system allows for understanding the differences between health and disease. Because healthcare resources remain limited, providing treatment that work are critical to establishing good healthcare outcomes. Understanding the methodology that provides the information needed to make these critical determinations serves as a critical success factor in managing and planning healthcare outcomes.

CHAPTER 9

Measuring Patient Satisfaction

INTRODUCTION TO MEASURING PATIENT SATISFACTION

In today's competitive and evolving healthcare delivery system, ongoing solicitation of feedback is a critical element in measuring healthcare outcomes from the patients' perspective. "No measure, no margin; no margin, no mission" reminds healthcare professionals that they must be able to measure a consumer's opinion of critical success factors or they will not remain an economically viable provider of healthcare delivery.

Gathering information about the quality of services provided by clinicians has never been more important (Gordon and Rehm, 1996). Clinicians are being held accountable for all aspects of healthcare delivery services by rising consumer expectations, by public and private healthcare purchasers, and by managed care plans responding to a competitive insurance market. Increasingly, the employers who purchase health benefits are becoming more reliant on systematic accountability for quality and cost of health care delivered to their employees. For example, managed care plans seek accreditation from the National

Committee on Quality Assurance (NCQA) to serve as the "Good Housekeeping" seal of approval to purchasers of healthcare benefits.

The development of the Health Plan Employer Data and Information Set (HEDIS) was a collaborative effort of the NCQA, health plan executives, and large national employer groups. HEDIS represents a core set of performance measures developed to assist employers/purchasers in defining the value of one managed care plan to another. In addition, HEDIS measures were designed as a system to hold managed care plans accountable for their performance. HEDIS also contains a performance measure which examines both members' access to clinical care and patient satisfaction. This measure includes related questions which ask the health plan to define their action plans for addressing these areas. Rather than setting benchmarks, HEDIS looks to see if the managed care plan has established its own set of standards. Then HEDIS asks how the actual scores of the panel clinicians credentialed by the plan compare with the plan's standards. HEDIS inquires about the following information: health plan performance data on overall member satisfaction, descriptions of the member satisfaction survey including a summary of results, and individual physician's performance related to patient satisfaction and access issues.

A major consideration of large employer groups and other major purchasers of healthcare delivery goods and services is that clinicians meet the expectations of patients—their employees. The real bottom line has to do with improving the health and well-being of patients and reducing their risk to illness and disease.

THE ASSESSMENT OF PATIENT SATISFACTION

In the most obvious sense, when any health care is provided by a healthcare professional to a patient, it is important to take into account of how that care is viewed and valued by the patient. According to Fitzpatrick (1997), the first half of the twentieth century was consumed by medicine's biomedical and technological approach to diagnosing and treating disease states and had significant indifference to patients' wishes and preferences for care. As the biopsychosocial approach (Engel, 1988) gained popularity within the medical establishment, healthcare delivery systems have sought to achieve a balance in services that are effective, scientific, and evidence-based while maintaining sensitivity to patients' needs and preferences.

Maxwell (1984) identified six dimensions under which the quality of modern medicine may be evaluated: access to care, relevance to need, effectiveness, equity, efficiency, and social acceptability. Social acceptability encompasses patient satisfaction. Often, these dimensions often have to be traded-off against each other. For example, the drive for cost-efficiency within the complexities of the delivery of health care to large numbers of patients may jeopardize satisfaction at the level of the individual patient. It is for this reason Fitzpatrick (1997) admonishes the healthcare delivery system to assess the impact of healthcare delivery services in terms of patient satisfaction as well as healthcare outcomes as a whole including morbidity, mortality, functionality, and quality of life.

The healthcare delivery system and its processes of care can influence patient satisfaction. Thus, patient satisfaction has become the subject of intense investigation in the healthcare delivery systems of developed countries (Fitzpatrick, 1997). Patient satisfaction is seen as an important indicator of the quality of health care. For this reason, all of the healthcare constituencies seek to obtain evidence of patients' views of quality of care received to use in the continuous process of monitoring and improving healthcare service delivery. Additionally health services research has grown enormously. Patient satisfaction measures are necessary in research context to provide valid and generalizable results from health research studies. Robust measures of patient satisfaction have been needed that could be used to examine alternative forms of providing health care in randomized or observational studies. Finally, measuring patient satisfaction contributes to other outcomes that are of great importance to purchasers and providers of healthcare services.

Studies have noted that patients who are dissatisfied with their care are less likely to reattend for further care (Weiss and Senf, 1990). Other studies have noted that dissatisfied patients are also less likely to comply with treatment regimens (Fitzpatrick and Hopkins, 1981). There is also evidence in the scientific literature that links lower levels of patient dissatisfaction with poorer health outcomes (Deyo and Diehl, 1986).

Patient satisfaction is considered to be a multi-dimensional construct. Fitzpatrick (1997) notes that most approaches to understanding patient satisfaction view patients' experiences include cognitive evaluations together with emotional reactions to their care. At a cognitive level, patients appraise the value of treatment received, and arrive at some positive, neutral, or negative response. Patients are capable of making quite complex and differentiated judgments of the quality of their care. Patients may hold distinct and independent views on how humanely they were treated and may also develop an opinion as to the cost-efficiency and accessibility of the care received within the context of the healthcare delivery system as a whole. Dimensions of patient satisfaction may include but are not limited to the following: humaneness, informativeness, quality, competence, access, cost, and attention to psychosocial issues.

MEASURING HUMANITY

Exploring the aspect of humanity in healthcare outcomes management and planning means assessing the social, psychological, and ethical acceptability of the way people are treated within the healthcare delivery system (Sinclair, 2000). The term humanity describes the quality of being civil, courteous, or obliging towards other people. It is characterized by sympathy with and consideration for others, especially patients who are receiving healthcare goods and services. Humanity also involves respect for dignity and autonomy of patients and a commitment to maximize the benefits obtained by healthcare services delivered to patients at the point of care while minimizing harm. It is not an unusual finding that patients are treated inhumanely by the healthcare delivery system. It may be an overt disregard for the sanctity of the patient–clinician relationship or it may be a covert action accepted as a cultural phenomenon repeated by many within the confines of a large, bureaucratic healthcare delivery system.

Assessing humanity involves a range of activities including handling patient complaints, monitoring standards of care, investigating claims of inhumanity, and assessing the impact of new interventions and changes in the healthcare delivery system. The following section is a synopsis of work produced by Donald Sinclair, MD, from the London School of Hygiene and Tropical Medicine (2000), that formally and thoroughly explores the quantitative and qualitative measurement of patient satisfaction from a biopsychosocial approach to healthcare delivery using humanity as the basis for understanding another dimension of healthcare outcomes management and planning.

HUMANITY AND PATIENT SATISFACTION

Inhumanity in health care often comes to the public's attention through various forms of press releases to the community-at-large. Gross negligence and carelessness resulting in undue suffering and death often makes front page news in local, regional, national, and world venues for all to see and hear. Cries from the public for reforms in healthcare delivery are often the result of such displays of inhumanity in the press.

What is considered as a right, entitlement, or expectation for every patient who receives healthcare delivery services from a humane perspective? There are four basic dimensions that make up humanity in the context of healthcare outcomes management and planning: autonomy, dignity, beneficence, and non-maleficence (Beauchamp and Childress, 1994). Autonomy is the dimension that enables people to exercise free will and the right to make choices about their actions and about what happens to them. From a healthcare perspective, autonomy suggests that patients should have the right to decide their own treatment, refuse treatment if they so desire, and be fully involved in all personal healthcare decisions. Dignity is the dimension that represents people being worthy of respect and indicates that everyone has the right to be treated with courtesy and consideration for his/her personal feelings. To accept this dimension, one must treat all people as equally valued. Beneficence is the dimension that has people striving to do good things for others. This obviously should be the motivation for all healthcare providers. For example, where there is a choice in healthcare intervention, it is usual to provide the intervention that is likely to provide the most benefits or best outcome to the patient. Finally, non-maleficence is the dimension of humanity that represents the principle of avoiding harm. Where there is a choice of healthcare intervention, the least harmful intervention to the patient that will still maximize the best outcome should be provided. It is certainly the hope that nobody would directly cause harm to a patient knowingly and maliciously (Sinclair, 2000).

Media coverage of inhumane situations or events is the most common way of bringing inhumanity to public attention. Patient complaints, investigative reports, or reports from special interest groups can trigger this publicity. Other sources of information regarding inhumane treatment of patients may come from the internal complaints system of a healthcare delivery organization, special reports or inquiries by public and private groups, and surveys and qualitative healthcare research. Gross inhumane treatment in health care is easy to imagine. For example, the deinstitutionalization of mental healthcare patients directly resulted from identifying gross negligence and inhumanity to patients on the psychiatric wards during the mid-twentieth century. However, there can be more subtle forms of inhumanity such as those inflicted by the organizational needs of large healthcare delivery systems, routine and mundane clinical care, and lack of consideration for the dignity of patients.

There are some limits to humanity and the treatment of patients within the healthcare delivery system. Just as patients have the right to receive humane clinical care, patients are also expected to attend their appointments, answer questions regarding their health and behavior honestly, and comply with agreed upon treatment action plans. However, there may be a conflict between the rights of individuals to expect humane care and the health needs of the population. For example, efficiency can conflict with humanity. While healthcare resource constraints, healthcare delivery systems must run services efficiently and maximize health gain for the largest number of people in the service population. The need for patient throughput at the point of care may limit the time available for the clinician–patient encounter and may jeopardize the quality of care delivered. Society may also have prevailing attitudes about the level of service provided to groups of people within the population such as the elderly, disabled, and mentally ill.

It is reasonable to assume that people who receive humane treatment within the healthcare delivery system will also be satisfied with the healthcare services they received. There is a separate consideration of satisfaction with the way health care is provided from the outcomes that are achieved with the same healthcare services. It is important to make the distinction here that for the purposes of understanding outcomes management and planning from a humanity perspective, measuring humanity will be taken to mean measuring patient satisfaction with the processes of care as they affect the dimensions of autonomy, dignity, beneficence, and non-maleficence. This involves assessing patients' experience of healthcare delivery, including the behavior of staff, the healthcare environment and the way in which patients are informed and empowered to participate in planning and managing their own treatment.

Whether patients complain or do not complain about their treatment within the healthcare delivery system, the individual query may not accurately represent the valid measurement of patient satisfaction. A lack of complaints regarding healthcare service delivery does not mean that the service is satisfactory. Sociodemographics and cultural norms play a large role in how people respond to questions about service. According to Fitzpatrick (1997), there are five main areas of healthcare experience which have a major impact on the amount of satisfaction expressed by patients: interpersonal skills of professionals, information given from health professionals, technical competence, the organization of health care, and time.

Interpersonal skills affect how well clinicians can interact with their patients and enable them to take a more active role in the clinician–patient relationship. A commitment to good interpersonal skills demonstrates a commitment to respecting patients' dignity. The way clinicians give information allows patients to be fully informed about the risks and benefits of the care they may or may not want to receive. This demonstrates a commitment to respect for patient autonomy. Technical competence refers to patient satisfaction with the clinician's ability to provide appropriate healthcare services. The education, training, and performance by the clinician at the point of care relates to the balance between beneficence and non-maleficence. The organization of the healthcare delivery system can affect all aspects of humanity. If patients feel that the system is overly bureaucratic, then they may perceive a lack of respect for both dignity and autonomy. Finally, time can affect autonomy and dignity. With the pressure to see more patients in less time, patients may begin to feel less valued as an individual and have less input into the decision-making process for their treatment action plan.

In summary, humanity involves treating people as individuals and respecting their rights of expression and self-determination. It also involves caring for people in a compassionate way and avoiding unnecessary suffering. There are four major dimensions of humanity identified in the process of measuring patient satisfaction: autonomy, dignity, beneficence, and non-maleficence (Beauchamp and Childress, 1994). When measuring patient satisfaction, one must consider which dimensions of humanity the interventions being evaluated will affect prior to measuring patient satisfaction. There are several different healthcare processes that have been shown to influence patient satisfaction: interpersonal skills of the clinician, information-giving by the clinician, technical competence, organization of healthcare delivery, and time (Fitzpatrick, 1997). The methodology for measuring patient satisfaction can be either by quantitative or qualitative processes.

QUANTITATIVE METHODS FOR MEASURING PATIENT SATISFACTION

Understanding humanity and how it is measured in terms of patient satisfaction with the processes of healthcare delivery has been discussed at length. It is possible to use quantitative methods, such as surveys, to measure patient satisfaction. Surveys are a form of evaluation based on the participants' own responses to a specific set of questions. The participants' are a representative sample of a selected population and information about them is gathered and analyzed systematically. Questions are carefully standardized so that they will provide data that can be quantitatively assessed. From a healthcare perspective, social surveys are defined as non-experimental studies of a population for the purpose of gaining information on specific aspects of health (Abramson, 1990).

Quantitative methods are most often used when it is known precisely which aspects of humanity (i.e., autonomy, dignity, beneficence, nonmaleficence) are to be measured. For example, assessing patient satisfaction with the way health information has been provided is what is going to be measured. Before the actual design of the survey begins, one may want to consider the following: specificity of the survey, location of the survey, timing of the survey, and content of the survey (Sinclair, 2000; Layte and Jenkinson, 1997). In determining the specificity of the survey, one must determine whether a narrow or broad definition of patient satisfaction is needed. For example, is a particular intervention the source of the health information or is it a more general assessment of health information delivered to the patient of interest? The location of the survey could be in any of the venues of the point of care: inpatient, outpatient, ancillary areas, etc. The timing of the survey is important because satisfaction can change with time. For example, patients may forget unpleasant experiences as an inpatient upon discharge home. In addition, satisfaction may change with one's health status. Finally, the content of the survey needs to be determined. What aspects of humanity are being investigated? Is the availability of healthcare information being investigated or is the environment or the relationships between people such as the clinician–patient relationship?

The Eleven Stages of Quantitative Survey Design

There are a number of steps to follow in designing a quantitative survey for assessing patient satisfaction (Layte and Jenkinson, 1997; McNeil,

1990). Stage 1 is an essential step in any research and begins with selecting a topic and reviewing the relevant scientific literature. Stage 2 develops a set of issues to be addressed by the survey. These issues are those aspects of humanity that have been chosen to be measured. For example, the survey may determine how well patients are empowered to play an active role in making decisions about their treatment. Stage 3 identifies the population to be surveyed. The population is defined in terms of its experience with the healthcare intervention that is being evaluated. Either the entire population affected must be surveyed or an appropriate sample of the population must be selected. Stage 4 is performing preliminary investigations. This may be as simple as asking a few patients and staff about their experiences with the aspect of patient satisfaction that is being studied. A qualitative study could also be performed during this stage. This stage is really only interested in identifying the relevant issues raised rather than in measuring the frequency of people's experiences. Stage 5 begins the draft of the questionnaire or selecting an available, standardized questionnaire. Questions are chosen to measure the relevant aspects of patient satisfaction. A decision as to how the questions are to be administered (self-completion vs. face-to-face) is required in this stage.

Choosing questions for the survey can be a very difficult process. Stone (1993) developed five criteria for selecting questions in a survey: appropriate, intelligible, unambiguous, unbiased, and omnicompetent. An appropriate question is one that asks the right thing. An intelligible question is one that is easily understood by the participant. An unambiguous question is one that asks only what the question is intended to and nothing else. An unbiased question covers the issues consistently for all healthcare interventions studied. Finally, an omnicompetent question is one that is able to record any response that the subject could make. The resources available to the researcher determine how the questionnaire will be administered. Obviously, interviewers are going to be more expensive than a self-completion survey. In addition, the subjects who are being surveyed will also determine the mode of administration. Highly technical questions may require interviewers to explain them to the participants. Certain topics may be too personal to discuss in the presence of an interviewer. Questions may be open—what did you like about the intervention?—or closed—did you like the intervention? Rating scales can be used to identify severity and frequency of feelings towards the intervention being measured.

Stage 6 is when the pilot study is performed. This stage can be very informative in the overall process of the study. Two groups of patients are recruited for this stage—one who has experienced the intervention being measured and one who has experienced an alternative or no intervention at all. Both groups of patients are asked to answer the draft questionnaire and to comment on the design and structure. Based on the responses, a determination is made as to whether the questions fulfill all of Stone's five criteria for survey questions. During this stage the questions for the final survey are being formalized. Stage 7 is the actual finalization of the questionnaire. It is during this stage that the questionnaire is determined to be valid, reliable, and reproducible.

At this point reliability and validity must be defined within the context of measuring patient satisfaction. Reliability refers to the ability of a questionnaire to produce consistent results over a period of time for the same population. Therefore, if the questionnaire is considered to be reliable, any change in the results is assumed to reflect a change in the amount of patient satisfaction. Validity describes the extent to which a questionnaire measures what the questionnaire was designed to measure, in this case patient satisfaction. There are several types of validity including face validity, content validity, criterion validity, and construct validity. Face validity describes whether the intended meaning of the questions in the questionnaire is obvious. Good face validity in a questionnaire means the questions are clear, unambiguous, and do not require much interpretation. Content validity describes whether the nature of the questions and their relative importance are appropriate to the purpose of the questionnaire. A questionnaire with good content validity should ask questions relevant to the aspect of patient satisfaction being studied. Criterion validity refers to the ability of the questionnaire to produce results that are compatible with other measurement techniques. In an ideal setting, one could test the questionnaire developed and implemented for measuring patient satisfaction against a widely accepted standardized questionnaire. However, most likely there is no standardized questionnaire available that measures the particular aspect of patient satisfaction under study. Finally, construct validity refers to the ability of the questionnaire to conform to expected hypotheses. For example, those individuals who have adequate insurance coverage for the healthcare intervention being studied are more apt to be satisfied with the process of having the procedure selected to be given to them than those who may not have adequate insurance coverage for the same procedure and had to pay out of pocket for a significant share of the cost, especially if the procedure was considered to be very costly.

Responsiveness relates to both reliability and validity in that it refers to the ability of the questionnaire to detect important changes in the patient. Responsiveness depends on the items that have been included in the questionnaire and their relative importance. For example, if one is interested in knowing which treatment protocol has the least number of side effects, the questionnaire should have questions that actually ask about the side effects of the treatment protocols. One would then weight the responses according to how much distress any given side effect caused the patients. Then, a change in side effects which results in a noticeable change in a patient's quality of life may be detected.

Stage 8 selects an appropriate sample of the population being studied. The individuals included in the sample who will receive the questionnaire should actually represent the population to which the results will be applied. Sampling refers to the process of identifying individuals for inclusion in the survey. Sampling may be either random or non-random. Random sampling aims to produce a group of individuals which is small enough to be surveyed within the available resources. However this group should still be large enough to represent all the major characteristics of the population from which it has been drawn. Random sampling requires the following:

- The definition of the sampling frame which is a list of all individuals eligible to be included
- Analysis of the data in the sampling frame to determine whether it really represents the population to be studied (e.g., age, gender, severity of illness, etc.)
- Estimation of the sample size

If there is some idea of the proportion of the population who are likely to be satisfied with the intervention, one can easily estimate the sample size using the following equation:

$$n = \pi (1-\pi) / [S.E. (p)]^2$$

where n = the sample size, π = proportion in the population with a particular attribute, and S.E. (p) = the smallest preferred standard error (Layte and Jenkinson, 1997).

Of course, simple equations like the above equation are of little use when the purpose of the survey is to find the prevalence of a particular aspect of patient satisfaction that is not yet known to the researcher before the survey is developed. Non-random sampling may be used when random sampling cannot be performed. For example, opportunistic sampling is a form of non-random sampling and refers to the process of including those individuals who are conveniently accessible. It may be the only practical technique if time and resources are limited. However, there is no reason to believe that the individuals selected represent the wider population. It may be necessary to compare a number of key attributes in the sample with those in the reference population to determine how representative the sample is.

Stage 9 is used to train interviewers, if necessary. If the survey requires interviewers, then they must be trained to ask the questions in a consistent manner to eliminate bias. Stage 10 is when the data is collected. The timing of the collection of the data may be very important. Bias may be a problem if individuals are surveyed a long time after they have experienced the healthcare intervention. Responses to all the questions of the questionnaire need to be coded in a fashion that facilitates analysis. The codes should distinguish clinically important responses. Stage 11 is the final stage where analysis of the data is performed and reports are written. This stage is important because decisions must be made as to how non-responses and missing data are to be explained. Allowances should be made for possible bias and confounding. Analyses should be performed by measuring the proportions of patients receiving each healthcare intervention who are satisfied with those evaluated aspects of their care. These proportions can then be compared using appropriate statistical techniques which are beyond the scope of this discussion.

In summary, quantitative methods of assessing patient satisfaction are appropriate when one knows precisely which aspects of humanity are selected to be evaluated. Surveys in the form of questionnaires have a rather complex process to be followed to ensure that the results of the questionnaire will be valid, reliable, and reproducible. There is the same need to avoid bias and confounding in surveys as in other study designs. If the aspects of humanity to be evaluated are not precisely known, then a qualitative methodology may be employed.

QUALITATIVE METHODS FOR MEASURING PATIENT SATISFACTION

When the aspects of humanity one wishes to evaluate are not known, it is not possible to design a quantitative survey to measure patient satisfaction. It is then necessary to employ a qualitative method. Qualitative methods allow for the exploration of reasons why people act in the way that they do, in this case to assess patient satisfaction with the processes of healthcare delivery.

Quantitative methods tell how often an event has occurred, and allow for the counting of numbers of people affected. Qualitative methods are based on observing what people do, exploring the way they interpret their experiences, and examining the impact that the research process has on their behavior. Qualitative methodology seeks to discover why individuals hold particular beliefs and why they perform particular actions. Qualitative methods also are concerned with how people behave and how social systems, such as healthcare delivery systems, operate. This methodology focuses on the individuals rather than on the diseases or clinical outcomes.

The techniques used in qualitative research are ideal for evaluating humanity when one is unable to decide in advance which aspects of humanity (i.e., autonomy, dignity, beneficence, non-maleficence) are to be measured. Sometimes qualitative methods are used to help plan quantitative studies. For example, one may wish to use a randomized control trial (RCT) to compare two healthcare interventions. One could use qualitative methodology to determine which healthcare outcomes are important to patients, and then design the RCT to measure these outcomes.

Qualitative methodology can explore issues or problems identified in quantitative studies. For example, a quantitative study may have identified patients who were dissatisfied with how clinicians provided information. One could use a qualitative survey to investigate the reasons for the failure to communicate between patient and clinician.

There are two types of qualitative methodologies useful in measuring patient satisfaction: observation and interviews. Observation techniques seek to examine what people do as well as what they say. Qualitative observation may be non-participant or participant. It may also be covert or overt. Non-participant observation describes the process of visiting one point of care where healthcare delivery services are provided and observing what the staff and patients do and say. For example, if one was interested in measuring patients' satisfaction with their experiences in an outpatient clinic, one would simply visit the clinic, sit down, and watch and listen to how people behave.

Participant observation describes the process where the researcher interacts with the subjects while they are going about their activities. In this technique, the observer not only observes what people do and say, but can ask questions of the subjects to help clarify observations. Continuing with the previous example, the only difference with using the participant observation technique would be that the researcher would ask the patients questions to clarify his observations of their behavior and communication in the outpatient clinic.

Covert observation refers to the situation where people being observed are unaware of the observer. Covert participant observation involves the researcher becoming part of the group (staff or patient) without allowing those being observed to know that they are being studied. Covert non-participant observation refers to a situation where the researcher simply watches without being noticed, most likely through a one way mirror. Obviously, covert research may raise some ethical considerations; however this approach may be justifiable in well-defined situations. Overt observation occurs when the subjects are aware that they are being observed.

Interviews differ from observation methodology because they involve specific communication between the researcher and the subjects' outside of the subjects' "normal" behavior (Ziebland and Wright, 1997). Interviews may be described according to their degree of structure. A highly structured interview may involve the researcher asking a set of predetermined questions in a predetermined order. A semi-structured interview may be no more than a simple conversation between the researcher and the subjects about a series of predetermined topics.

Interviews may be performed on a one-on-one basis or in a group setting. Focus groups are a form of a group interview. A focus group comprises between six and twelve participants and a facilitator. The participants often share similar characteristics, such as a clinical diagnosis or sociodemographic type. The facilitator guides the group through a series of predetermined topics that the researcher wants discussed in a permissive, non-threatening environment (Krueger, 1994). In this form of group discussion, participants may feel able to express their opinions better than in a one-on-one interview. For example, once a participant expresses dissatisfaction about a particular clinical process, then others in the group may feel more at ease to express a similar dissatisfaction. The focus group may also allow the researcher to understand how knowledge and opinions are formed through social interaction.

A nominal group is similar to a focus group but concentrates on only one topic to allow for more structure to the format of discussion. Each patient's views are then grouped when similar and discussed by the whole group. They are then rank ordered by high to low importance by the entire group (Moore, 1994). Nominal group technique is useful in identifying problems, exploring solutions, and establishing priorities.

Interviews, as a qualitative methodology used in social surveys, can be used rather effectively in healthcare outcomes management and planning (Ziebland and Wright, 1997). Interviews can help determine the views and opinions of the public, healthcare consumers, clinicians, and all healthcare constituencies. Interviews can explore the views of various participants in a research area. This technique gathers ideas and generates hypotheses for use in quantitative social survey research. Interviews can investigate sensitive topics and allow for better understanding of the meaning behind people's experiences and behaviors within a healthcare delivery system. When dealing with sensitive topics, semi-structured interviews allow subjects to control the discussion and approach the topic in their own way and therefore may result in a better response. Focus groups can also handle sensitive topics. If all the members of the focus group consider themselves to have similar interests and vulnerabilities, they may give each other the confidence to discuss such private and personal topics. Interviews also allow for the exploration of issues revealed by quantitative social surveys.

Interviews can also help to understand the risks involved in a variety of healthcare interventions and situations. This is called critical incident analysis (Sinclair, 2000). Critical incident analysis is a form of case-study and involves reviewing situations where disasters have occurred or have been narrowly avoided. Interviews are conducted with all the individuals involved in the disaster and all relevant information is examined. This process aims to identify critical points in the decision-making process where changes can be made to prevent the situation from being repeated in the future.

Validity in qualitative research is equally as important as it is in quantitative research. The validity of the qualitative methodology used depends on the following factors: study design, sampling method, and data collection. In the study design of qualitative social surveys, it is important that qualitative methods be used for qualitative questions. For example, a qualitative question would take the following form, "How do patients perceive their healthcare processes?" The methods must be appropriate to the questions. For certain topics, group interviews may be better than individual sessions. Some information may be only revealed by one of the techniques of observation previously discussed.

The sampling method used in qualitative research is much different than what is used in quantitative research. Rather than sampling a portion of the population to represent the entire population, qualitative sampling seeks to find a group of people that will provide a broad range of views and opinions. Data collection in qualitative research is concerned with obtaining the true, unbiased views of subjects. Interviewers must be carefully trained to avoid prejudicing the responses obtained from the participants of the study.

Analysis of qualitative data is also quite different from that of quantitative research (Ziebland and Wright, 1997). When coding qualitative data, the researcher should aim to identify all items of data that are present in the observations or in the records of the interviews. One should then attempt to determine which items are related to one another to detect a pattern within the responses. For example, if one is measuring patient satisfaction with the way health information has been given to the participants of the study, themes may emerge as patterns from their responses such as lack of staff approachability, appearance of staff indifference to the patients, and overuse of medical jargon during clinician–patient interaction. Textual analysis is a process of searching textual data for specific words or phrases. The aim is to identify key concepts present in the material and to discover the relationships between them. The key words and phrases are detected by eye or computer and coded. Their context may be deduced from the surrounding text acquired from the interviewing process.

Determining the validity of the data is a key process during the analysis phase. Researchers employ several techniques in order to verify the data. The data can be searched for disconfirming evidence or inconsistencies. A process called triangulation can also be used. This process uses different sources of data or different methods to examine the same question. If the results are similar, supporting evidence for their validity emerges.

Finally, the researcher may review the findings with one of the original participants of the study. This is called respondent validation and it may enable the researcher to obtain a deeper understanding both of the concepts studied and their relationships.

Reporting the findings of any qualitative study, and specifically reporting the humanity aspects of a healthcare intervention requires the following:

1. Explaining the choice of which particular aspects of patient satisfaction to assess, and their relevance to the healthcare intervention(s) or clinical care processes that are being evaluated.
2. Describing the methodology employed in the study and explaining why the methodology was chosen.
3. Describing the results of the study and the reasons the researcher believes the data is valid.
4. Applying the results of the study to the healthcare interventions lor clinical processes that are being evaluated (Ziebland and Wright, 1997).

In summary, qualitative methods used in social surveys are concerned with how people behave and how social systems operate in a natural context. They may be used to ask questions about how or why people behave in particular ways. They can also be used to investigate people's beliefs and their reasons for having these beliefs. Qualitative methods are ideal for evaluating patient satisfaction when the most important aspects of satisfaction can not be determined in advance. Qualitative techniques include observation and interviewing, and require a systematic process to follow that is similar to that of quantitative research. Once the data has been obtained, analyzing the data requires the process of validation to determine if the data truly reflects the question posed by the researcher.

CONCLUSION

Rising healthcare consumer's expectations are holding clinicians more accountable for all healthcare services being delivered today. Measuring patient satisfaction is a critical element in measuring healthcare outcomes. Patient satisfaction and loyalty are critical success factors for the economic viability for all providers of healthcare services today.

Measuring Cost Effectiveness

INTRODUCTION TO HEALTHCARE ECONOMICS

In order to fully appreciate the magnitude of determining cost effectiveness in healthcare outcomes management and planning, a short primer on healthcare economics is required. Many professional programs do not teach the basic concepts and theories of healthcare economics as part of the medical school curriculum in the applied medical sciences. Often both clinicians and administrators realize the importance that healthcare economics plays in the delivery of healthcare goods and services only during the practical experience.

When beginning to explore the basic concepts and theories of healthcare economics, one question arises: "Why do individual patients and the community-at-large demand healthcare goods and services?" Several factors have been identified to answer this question. First, the United States has been experiencing changes in the age structure of the general population for several decades. People are generally living longer, but not necessarily healthier, with adequate functionality and an expressed excellent quality of life. Second, as real and disposable income has increased, consumers of healthcare delivery goods and services have developed higher expectations with respects to healthcare outcomes (i.e., access, quality, service, satisfaction, value, etc.). Finally, improvements in healthcare technology and the growth of medical informatics as a separate discipline within the applied medical sciences have led to an increased range of healthcare interventions. As the demand for healthcare goods and services continues to change and evolve within the next few decades, the need for professional healthcare administrators and clinicians to better understand the basic concepts and theories of healthcare economics becomes more critical.

Health economics (Mills and Gilson, 1988) may be broadly defined as the application of the theories, concepts and techniques of economics to the healthcare delivery system. Several key areas of interest within the discipline of applied medical sciences include:

- The allocation of resources (i.e., land, labor, capital) between various health promoting activities
- The quantity of resources used in healthcare delivery
- The administrative organization and funding of healthcare institutions
- The efficiency with which healthcare resources are allocated and used for clinical and administrative healthcare delivery
- The effects of preventive, curative, and rehabilitative healthcare services on individual utility and societal welfare

The overall aim of healthcare economics is to inform the healthcare constituencies so that choices for allocating and using healthcare goods and services maximize the benefits and outcomes to the applicable population and individuals. Healthcare economics is *not* about saving money within the healthcare delivery system. It is about doing the right thing, at the right amount, in the right way, at the right time. If you take care of people, the financials will take care of themselves.

Healthcare economics may be examined at both a macro and micro level of attention. Macroeconomics deals with the behavior of the overall healthcare economy. It focuses on the assessment of income, employment, productivity, and healthcare expenditures on a local, regional, national, or global level. Microeconomics deals with the behavior of individual households and the principles and practices of supply and demand. Within the realm of supply and demand, elasticity refers to the demand for healthcare goods and services that change concomitantly with price. For example, if health care were considered to be elastic, as the price of prescription drugs increases, the demand for these prescription drugs should decrease. Consequently, the supply increases at the retail pharmacy. However, health care is considered to be inelastic in that supply and demand for goods and services respond slightly or not at all to changes in price. For example, the price for insulin syringes increases; the demand remains stable and the supply is unchanged because diabetic patients still require syringes to inject insulin and they will find a way to pay for them regardless of price increase.

Because healthcare demand is inelastic, an important issue is raised. Brown et al. (2005) question how healthcare inflation can be reduced to a reasonable level given the demand for healthcare delivery goods and services is inelastic and the "normal" market forces of supply and demand do not readily apply. The answer lies within the need to maximize the healthcare "value" received from the resources used based on the healthcare dollars expended.

A closer look into the macroeconomics of healthcare delivery in the United States is required (Brown et al., 2005). There are some basic U.S. healthcare economic indicators that must be explained including the annual healthcare expenditure, the rate of healthcare inflation, the per capita healthcare expenditure, and the distribution of healthcare expenditures.

The annual healthcare expenditure in the United States, according to the Centers for Medicare and Medicaid Services (CMS) formerly known as the Health Care Financing Administration or HCFA (CMS, 2005; Brown et al., 2005), in 1970 was $73.1 billion dollars or approximately 7 percent of the gross domestic product (GDP). Adjustment of the 1970 expenditure for general inflation (established to be 5 percent) yields an expenditure of $356 billion dollars in year 2004. Estimated total healthcare expenditures in 2004 according to CMS are $1.773 trillion dollars or approximately 15.3 percent of the GDP. Thus, the total healthcare expenditure grew at a rate five times that expected with general inflation from 1970 to 2004. The annual healthcare expenditure in the United States is estimated to rise to $2.639 trillion dollars or 16.8 percent of the GDP by 2010.

The rate of healthcare inflation in the United States determined by measuring total healthcare expenditures, according to CMS (CMS, 2005; Brown et al., 2005), rose at an annual rate of 10 percent during a 30 year period from 1970 to 1999. During this time period, the general rate of inflation was 5 percent. If the rate of healthcare inflation continues at a rate of 10 percent for total healthcare expenditures, by 2010 the annual total healthcare expenditure amount will be $3.4 trillion dollars, or 20.4 percent of the GDP. This is much higher than the CMS estimated total healthcare expenditure amount of $2.6 trillion dollars, or 16.8 percent of the GDP.

The per capita healthcare expenditure is the amount spent on each person for healthcare services in the United States per year. In 1970, the per capita healthcare expenditure was $341 dollars. This amount is estimated (CMS, 2005; Brown et al., 2005) to be $6,126 in non-inflation adjusted nominal dollars in 2004, and is expected to rise to $8,704 nominal dollars by the year 2010. Adjusting for the rate of general inflation, according to the consumer price index the real dollar expenditure in 1970 dollars equates to $1,662 in 2004. Therefore, the data show a 3.7 times ($6,126/$1,662) increase in per capita expenditures above inflation over the past three decades. Therefore, the inflation-adjusted healthcare expenditure for the average U.S. citizen in 2004 is 3.7 times the amount expended for healthcare services in 1970. As Americans are living longer and with more chronic diseases in the age group of persons greater than 65 years old, the per capita expenditures on average can be as high as $16,000 dollars among persons over the age of 85 (Brown et al., 2005).

The United States' distribution of healthcare expenditures is a long list of healthcare providers who receive payment for healthcare delivery services rendered. The top three on this list include payments to physicians, payments to hospitals, and payments for prescription drugs. In 1970, payments to physicians accounted for 19 percent of healthcare expenditures, while hospital payments and payments for prescription drugs accounted for 38 percent and 8 percent respectively (CMS, 2005; Brown et al., 2005). As the primary point of care shifted from the inpatient hospital venue to outpatient venues (i.e., physician offices, ambulatory surgical, and medical venues, etc.) in 2000, payments to physicians increased to 22 percent, hospital payments decreased to 28 percent, and prescription drug payments increased to 9 percent. It is estimated that by 2010, the distribution of healthcare expenditures will change again with physician, hospital and prescription drug payments at 21 percent, 28 percent, and 14 percent respectively. As of 2003, physician payments were 21.8 percent, hospital payments were 30.4 percent, prescription drugs were 11 percent, administrative healthcare costs were 6.7 percent, research costs were 1.6 percent, and nursing home care accounted for 6.5 percent of the healthcare dollar (Brown et al., 2005).

Approximately 45 percent of healthcare costs are publicly funded while the other 55 percent is funded by the private sector. There are two large publicly funded healthcare programs in the United States today.

Medicare, which primarily covers senior citizens over the age of 65, disabled citizens under the age of 65, and people with end-stage renal disease requiring dialysis or kidney transplant; and Medicaid, which is a federal-state collaboration covering groups among the economically disadvantaged including children, pregnant women, adults in families with dependent children, individuals with disabilities and/or over the age of 65, and qualified individuals needing nursing home care. The importance of the Medicare system of payment is that it is the most standardized healthcare payment system in the United States today. While all healthcare third party insurers in the United States have complicated reimbursement systems, the great majority are based upon the Medicare system. This factor makes Medicare the best payment system to use for healthcare economic analysis. Medicare does alter payments for most healthcare interventions to account for geographic differences in costs. However, the average Medicare payment across the United States is the best for most economic analyses (Brown et al., 2005).

Healthcare dollars should be spent for the highest return possible in terms of improving individual and population healthcare outcomes such as morbidity, mortality, functionality, patient satisfaction, and quality of life. A data and information system (preferably electronically based) that allows for the highest return on investment for the healthcare dollars expended is required to achieve this goal. The fact that improving quality of life, functionality, and an overall sense of health and well-being also indirectly increases the productivity of the American population cannot be overestimated (Brown et al., 2005). This is a critical economic factor because improving worker productivity enables the general economy to grow positively. Improved productivity also contributes to the gross domestic product by allowing more goods and services to be available for consumption without accompanying inflation. It is evident to many that there are few factors (other than a healthy lifestyle) that contribute more to increasing individual productivity in all aspects of one's life.

EVIDENCE-BASED MEDICINE

Traditionally, the practice of clinical medicine has been based on principles and practices that have their origins in pathophysiology, biochemistry, genetics, deductive reasoning, and clinical experience (Rafuse, 1994). Most recently, healthcare constituencies (see Table 1-1) have demanded that the clinical delivery of healthcare goods and services be scientifically validated and reliable while producing favorable clinical, financial, and functional outcomes with high patient satisfaction scores. The recent development of evidence-based medicine (EBM) represents the philosophy that clinical medical practices should be based on the most valid, reliable, and reproducible scientific and clinical data and information available.

According to the principles and practices of EBM (Rafuse, 1994), any medical or surgical intervention should be based on scientific and/or clinical research that uses a valid, reliable, and reproducible methodology. From a practical perspective, EBM incorporates the latest scientific and clinical research into the delivery of healthcare goods and services at the point of care. Evidence-based medicine leverages a rapidly expanding global, scientific, and clinical database with state-of-the-art medical informatics capabilities for communicating in a real time manner that can be accessed instantaneously at the point of care during the clinician–patient encounter. The challenge that remains is to determine the data and information that is scientifically and clinically relevant, valid, and reliable and that will produce favorable healthcare outcomes for both individuals and the community-at-large.

Evidence-based medicine forms the basis for a problem-solving approach to clinical issues. Within a conceptual, scientific framework that has been used by clinicians in an ever-changing healthcare delivery system, EBM requires the careful gathering of data and information, processing what has been gathered, and attempting to use the data and information that is most important, relevant, and useful in caring for patients (Brown et al., 2005). Unfortunately, many clinicians remain unable to adequately apply the evidence of clinical research studies at the point of care. It has been estimated that from 1948 through 1994, the total sum of healthcare knowledge has increased 1342 times (Freitas, 2005). Obviously, the informatics explosion of the Internet and the proliferation of the personal computer has greatly influenced this increase.

According to Freitas (2005), the total sum of medical information now doubles in approximately three and one-half years. Continuing medical education requirements and the professional educational years requires clinicians to learn new data and information at an alarming pace and update criteria for clinical care regularly. These new clinical results change the standards of clinical care within the healthcare delivery system on a real-time basis. It is the hope that EBM will lead to improved healthcare outcomes management and planning. However, this can only happen if the clinicians embrace new point of care technology and medical informatics, which will improve the efficacy and effectiveness of the clinicians' ability to gather, store, process, and disseminate new, valid, and reliable scientific and clinical data and information.

The differentiation of the level of evidence for medical and surgical healthcare interventions is a complex process. Rather than blindly accepting a scientific clinical report at face value, clinicians must be able to quickly discern whether a negative study is underpowered, the important difference between relative risk reduction and absolute risk reduction, and the meaning of numbers to treat patients (Brown et al., 2005). Clinicians today must embrace and engage in EBM at the point of care to facilitate the healthcare delivery of high quality, cost-efficient, easily accessible, service-oriented, and customer-focused healthcare.

VALUE-BASED MEDICINE

Value-based medicine (VBM) according to Brown et al. (2005) takes evidence-based medicine (EBM) to a higher level. Value-based medicine incorporates all patient-perceived quality of life variables associated with a healthcare intervention. This allows for a more accurate measure of overall worth of a particular healthcare intervention than one obtained solely by primary evidence-based healthcare outcomes management and planning. Consequently, clinicians can deliver the highest quality, most cost-effective clinical care and receive a better understanding of the patient-perceived value.

Understanding the needs of patients from their perspective requires the healthcare delivery system to accept the following assumptions:

- Patients perceive their healthcare demands as what they believe they need to achieve to be healthy and well
- As a patient they are willing to accept whatever it will cost for them to be healthy and well
- As a patient they have the means and they are willing to spend out of pocket what it will cost to be healthy.

Evidence-based medicine is the scientific and clinical practice of medicine at the point of care based on the most accurate, valid, reliable, and reproducible medical data and information. Value-based medicine is the clinical practice of medicine based on the patient-perceived value conferred by a medical or surgical intervention (Brown et al., 2005). Value-based medicine takes the best EBM data and information and converts these data into value form. Value-based medicine also permits the comparison between the values conferred by the healthcare intervention to the healthcare resources expended on that particular intervention. Utility analysis is the process that allows the conversion of EBM data and information to VBM data and information. Cost-utility analysis is the process that further integrates the cost associated with the healthcare intervention. Cost-utility analysis according to Brown et al. (2005) is the instrument by which nearly all healthcare interventions are measured in terms of cost, evidence, and value providing a cost effective ratio for each intervention. This will ultimately lead to the creation of a comprehensive VBM database.

Value-based medicine takes disparate EBM data and information and converts it into patient-perceived value using a common healthcare outcome measure. This value conferred by healthcare interventions may then be compared on a common scale for almost every healthcare intervention available to patients today. Specifically, clinicians report EBM healthcare outcomes in terms of numbers. For example, coronary artery bypass improves the cardiac ejection fraction from 45 percent to the normal range of function between 50 percent and 65 percent. Another example is when cataract surgery improves the patient's visual function from 20/80 to 20/20.

Value-based medicine forces healthcare delivery to examine the EBM data and information from the patients' perspective by asking additional questions. For example:

- what is the patient-perceived value of coronary artery bypass surgery or cataract surgery from a functional and quality of life perspective (i.e., will the patient have improved walking distance after coronary artery bypass surgery or will the patient have improved night vision after the cataract surgery)?
- How can two such dissimilar healthcare interventions be compared in value from the patients' perspective?

THE MANAGEMENT OF VALUE

According to Brown et al. (2005), the value conferred by any healthcare intervention is measured by quantifying the improvement or maintenance it confers in terms of quality or length of life. An objective measure of value, standardized for all healthcare interventions, is required for determining cost-utility analysis. An objective value for all healthcare interventions provides the most accurate measurement of patient-perceived value of a healthcare intervention, the means to compare all healthcare interventions on the same scale, and a measure that may be combined with the cost of a healthcare intervention to arrive at a cost-utility ratio. The cost-utility ratio creates a single, quantifiable number for comparing healthcare interventions based on perceived patient-value and cost considerations to the healthcare delivery system.

Utility analysis is the primary tool used today in healthcare outcomes management and planning to measure the quality of life associated with a health or disease state from the patients' perspective. This type of analysis serves as the basis for developing a data repository capable of serving as the foundation for VBM. In health care today, there is a well-developed sequence for acquiring data and information and converting it into a knowledge-based format that is value-based in its content (Brown et al., 2005).

Evidence-based medicine begins the sequence of events leading to VBM. EBM healthcare intervention data and information is then converted to patient-perceived VBM data and information. Finally, cost-utility analysis combines the patient-perceived value of the healthcare intervention with the costs associated with a particular healthcare intervention to create a VBM database. The value conferred by a particular healthcare intervention and the cost-utility ratio associated with that healthcare intervention are the two most important healthcare outcomes in VBM.

COST-UTILITY ANALYSIS

Cost-utility analysis refers to a type of economic analysis whereby a healthcare outcome measures the healthcare resources (in U.S. dollars) expended for the value (i.e., improvement in quality or length of life) conferred by a healthcare intervention (Drummond et al., 1999). The healthcare outcome measure is the U.S. dollars expended for a quality-adjusted life-year gained ($/QALY). By definition, the number of QALYs gained from a particular healthcare intervention equals the utility value gained from the healthcare intervention, multiplied by the duration of the benefit in years. For example, a gain in utility of 0.5 for 4 years equals 2 QALYs gained.

Cost-effectiveness analysis refers to a type of healthcare economic analysis with a healthcare outcome measuring the healthcare resources (in U.S. dollars) expended per year of life gained or per year of good vision gained, or per year of good walking gained and so on (Brown et al., 2005). There is a clear distinction between *cost-utility analysis* and *cost-effectiveness analysis*. However, it is important to note here that cost-effectiveness analysis is the conventional term used in the peer-reviewed medical literature to describe both types of healthcare economic analysis. Cost-utility analysis is the more sophisticated form of healthcare economic analysis because it provides an objective measure of the "value" of healthcare interventions. Cost-utility analysis provides all healthcare constituencies with the value of healthcare goods and services provided and received by patients for the dollars expended.

According to Brown et al. (2005), healthcare constituencies commonly perceive the healthcare delivery system they are a part of in terms of rationing healthcare goods and services measured by cost-effectiveness and quality standards. Value-based medicine is not a form of healthcare delivery that rations services to patients at the point of care. Rather, value-based medicine communicates the healthcare interventions identified to have substantial value and those healthcare interventions that are of negligible value, of no value, or of harm to patients. If a healthcare intervention is costly but significantly improves healthcare outcomes for patients, it is cost-effective. If a healthcare intervention does not improve healthcare outcomes, then it is not cost-effective at any price.

Value-based medicine integrates all of the increments or decrements in quality of life associated with a particular healthcare intervention. It takes EBM healthcare outcomes and adds quality and length-of-life outcomes to the equation, along with issues of cost and healthcare resource use to demonstrate the value of healthcare interventions to patients. Therefore, the VBM information system improves the total quality of healthcare delivery and improves the efficient expending of limited healthcare resources. It is an issue of appropriate allocation of healthcare resources, not one of creating more healthcare resources. The major goal of VBM is to promote what is best for the patient using clinical services point of care.

THE BENEFITS OF VALUE-BASED MEDICINE

The benefits of VBM may be viewed from three perspectives: the patient, the clinician, and the community-at-large. At the present time, patients do not have a standardized source of information to provide them with reports on the value of a particular healthcare intervention. Often, it is word-of-mouth from other patients and their families who experienced a particular healthcare intervention who report their healthcare outcomes to others. This may or may not influence whether another patient will agree to experience the same healthcare intervention.

Value-based medicine proposes a standardized format for patients to evaluate treatment options using the opinions of other patients who have lived with and been treated for similar disease states. The VBM database would compile information on all medical, surgical, and pharmaceutical interventions. Again, at the present time, no such database exists in any healthcare delivery system at any level—local, regional, national, or global. Value-based medicine may be able to discern an overall negative or neutral healthcare outcome for a particular healthcare intervention when these healthcare outcomes are difficult to differentiate from EBM data and information alone. Patients will become empowered to seek alternative opinions from other clinicians, select an alternative healthcare intervention, or decide whether to let the disease run its natural course.

The quality and length-of-life variables addressed by VBM may dramatically improve the value of a particular healthcare intervention, decrease the value of a particular healthcare intervention, or place a particular healthcare intervention into a potentially harmful category. Most important is that the value conferred on a particular healthcare intervention be the most accurate, valid, reliable, and reproducible data and information for decision making because it is obtained using the preferences of other patients with similar clinical conditions. Value-based medicine allows patients to potentially receive the highest quality of clinical healthcare because VBM evaluates the worth of a healthcare intervention much better than EBM data and information alone.

Clinicians who deliver healthcare goods and services to patients will also benefit from VBM because they will develop a better perception of the actual value healthcare interventions convey to their patients at the point of care. In addition, all clinicians must access services in a healthcare delivery system as patients, and they too will benefit from the VBM database about the value of a particular healthcare intervention. Brown et al. (2005) believe when all the benefits and adverse effects associated with healthcare interventions are included in the overall equation in a VBM database, clinicians will be surprised that the overall value conferred is greater or less than they had previously believed.

The community-at-large will also benefit from VBM. As the costs of healthcare delivery continue to grow at a rate almost double that of general inflation (CMS, 2005; Brown et al., 2005), decisions regarding healthcare resource allocations must be made by all the healthcare constituencies. Value-based medicine will allow the most efficacious use of healthcare resources to help most people receive the highest quality of healthcare delivery possible for the resources expended. The most efficient use of healthcare resources is a critical factor for the United States to remain in a globally influential position with respects to healthcare delivery. Identification of healthcare interventions that are not cost-effective will allow the community-at-large to have input with healthcare policy-makers and clinicians as the future use of these healthcare interventions. If a particular healthcare intervention is identified as not being cost-effective, options that can bring a treatment into the range of cost-effectiveness should be considered. These options include improving the efficacy and effectiveness of the treatment, decreasing the associated costs of using the treatment, and/or altering the adverse effects by modifying healthcare interventions. For VBM to rise to the forefront and have all the healthcare constituencies recognize its importance, healthcare economic analysis must become methodologically stable, valid, reliable, and reproducible from academia to the point of care.

BARRIERS TO ENTRY FOR VALUE-BASED MEDICINE

Value-based medicine concepts and theories are not new to healthcare delivery. Klarman et al. (1968) were the first to describe the quality adjusted life year (QALY) in the peer-reviewed scientific literature almost 40 years ago. Weinstein and Stasson (1977) described cost-effectiveness analysis (the present day cost-utility analysis) almost 30 years ago and Sinclair et al. (1981) introduced the term cost-utility analysis in the peer-reviewed medical literature in 1981.

Lack of standardization in the evaluation process poses a barrier in performing cost-utility analysis as the primary measurement of VBM. Healthcare economic analysis is not an exact science and there is a wide variation in methodology used by analysts in this field. According to Brown et al. (2005), a healthcare economic analysis by definition is a multidisciplinary study design requiring inputs from the fields of clinical knowledge, epidemiology, economics, public policy, mathematics, and business. Therefore, analysts from the different disciplines bring different knowledge sets to their individual study designs and lack knowledge in other critical areas needed for a comprehensive healthcare economic evaluation.

Inconsistent study designs have become problematic due to methodological issues of controversy such as the decision perspective, the instruments used for measuring quality of life, the cost factor, and the rate used to account for the time preference (i.e., net present value or NPV) of money used in the analysis. Standardization of cost-utility analysis input variables will allow cost-utility analysis to be more broadly applied at all levels of healthcare policy decision making.

The guidelines currently used most often in cost-utility analysis are those developed by the Panel for Cost-Effectiveness in Health and Medicine during 1996 (Gold et al., 1996). The Panel for Cost-Effectiveness in Health and Medicine is a group organized by the United States Public Health Service to set standards of methodological practices for healthcare economic analysts. Some of the panel's recommendations include the use of preferences in cost-utility analysis, the performance of reference case (i.e., the average person with average variables associated with a health or disease state) analysis, discounting costs and outcomes at a 3 percent annual rate, and the use of sensitivity analysis. Despite a comprehensive academic treatise on cost-utility analysis, Brown et al. (2005) suggest there has been little effect on public policy and healthcare resource allocation in the United States. A detailed analysis as to the reasons why Brown feels the panel's recommendations are ineffective are discussed in their book (Brown et al., 2005).

VBM has not been widely incorporated into healthcare economic analysis because standard cost-utility input variables are lacking at the point of care. Other deterrents include the complexity of the subject; the lack of a standardized treatment for comorbid health and disease states; the lack of a standardized, preference-based, quality of life database; the fact that VBM may run counter to the interests of select healthcare constituencies; and the perception that VBM may lead to healthcare rationing rather than appropriate healthcare resource allocation (Brown et al., 2005).

There are healthcare interventions that provide minimal or no value to patients, clinicians, and the community-at-large. These healthcare interventions may actually be harmful to patients. VBM is a "antira-tioning" mechanism that allows for the appropriate allocation of health-care resources that bring the most value for the most patients at the point of care. Finally, all healthcare constituencies will embrace the concepts, theories, and applications of VBM in healthcare delivery because it allows patient input at the point of care in the form of preferences (measured as scales of time tradeoff, willingness to pay, functionality, and quality of life) for health and disease states and healthcare interventions to be included in treatment protocols, it improves the quality, cost, access and service of healthcare delivery at the point of care, and maximizes the effi-cacy, effectiveness, and efficiency of the allocation of valuable healthcare resources to be used a the point of care (Brown et al., 2005).

HEALTHCARE ECONOMICS AND ITS CONTRIBUTION TO OUTCOMES MANAGEMENT AND PLANNING

Before completing the discourse on healthcare economic analysis and measuring cost-effectiveness, it is important to review healthcare econom-ics as a scientific discipline, establish a framework for understanding all relevant areas within this discipline, and identify the contribution that healthcare economics has made to outcomes management and planning.

Healthcare economics is the applied scientific discipline of how all healthcare constituencies choose—with or without the use of money—to employ scarce, productive healthcare resources that could be used alterna-tively elsewhere and to produce and distribute healthcare goods and serv-ices for consumption on both a small or large scale, now or in the future. Healthcare economics also analyzes the costs and benefits of improving the distribution of valuable healthcare resources among the population. Healthcare economics applies to all healthcare activities where scarcity exists and choices exist related to the allocation of these resources. In summation, healthcare economics is the study of scarcity of healthcare resources and the judicious allocation of these resources in the healthcare delivery system (Mills and Gilson, 1988).

How does the applied scientific discipline of healthcare economics apply to healthcare outcomes management and planning? Before answer-ing this question, a model or framework of healthcare economics is required to fully explore all the subdisciplines of healthcare economics as they apply first to scarcity and allocation of resources and then second, to healthcare outcomes management and planning (Lee and Mills, 1983). To begin,

1. The influences of health must be determined by exploring occupational hazards, consumption patterns, education, income, and other biopsychosocial areas of interest.
2. Second, the value of health and the quantification of this value must be determined using functionality scales, health status indices, and other biopsychosocial surveys. Particular attention must be paid to the validity and reliability of these measuring tools.
3. Third, the influences of demand by healthcare consumers for the scarce healthcare resources must be determined. Time, access, quality, price, and behavior all influence individual and population demand for healthcare resources.
4. Fourth, the characteristics of the supply of scarce healthcare resources must be determined. Costs of production, mix of inputs, nature of the marketplace, and payment mechanisms all determine the characteristics of the supply side of healthcare economics.
5. Fifth, the costs and consequences of complimentary or alternative healthcare interventions must be considered to determine whether they improve or impair healthcare delivery at the point of care.
6. Sixth, the results of the interplay between the supply and demand of scarce healthcare services must be examined in terms of expended dollars, price, time, access, service, and allocation.
7. Seventh, the different ways of financing and organizing the healthcare delivery system must be delineated in terms of efficacy, effectiveness, efficiency, humanity, and equity.
8. Finally, the mechanisms that are in place (strategic planning, budgeting, regulations, etc.) within healthcare delivery systems must be identified. This identification process achieves the measurable objectives used to determine success and the appropriate allocation of scarce healthcare resources.

Healthcare outcomes management and planning is really about making rational choices in allocating scarce healthcare resources so that future goals of good health and well-being in the population can be achieved. As discussed previously, healthcare economics and outcomes management and planning have a definite affinity for one another. The nature and level of a country's economic development is a major determinant of the health status of its populace and it is associated with the level of healthcare delivery a country can support both publicly and privately.

Healthcare outcomes management and planning is strongly influenced by macroeconomic considerations of inflation, the consumer price index, employment, and the production of healthcare goods and services. The health and well-being of a population at any level may itself influence economic progress and healthcare outcomes management and planning. Healthcare delivery programs in the form of direct and indirect healthcare services have become part of a comprehensive strategy aimed at improving the biopsychosocial welfare of its demanding population. This strategy demands healthcare programs that improve healthcare outcomes most effectively and efficiently, such as clinical preventive services, health counseling, public health initiatives, disease state management, and others.

The United States, as described earlier, has a healthcare inflation rate that is double that of the general inflation rate with no real end in sight (CMS, 2005; Brown et al., 2005). Healthcare delivery systems are actively seeking ways of containing costs, increasing efficiency, and tapping additional resources. The principles and practices of healthcare economics become vital for these healthcare delivery systems. They help improve the allocation of scarce healthcare resources, increase the efficiency of healthcare services delivered at the point of care, identify more cost-effective technologies, and evaluate alternative sources of health finance. Improvement of healthcare outcomes clinically, financially, functionally, and satisfactorily is the ultimate goal of making difficult choices based on understanding a model or framework of healthcare economics presented earlier. As healthcare delivery progresses into the future, healthcare economic analysis is the primary measure of whether healthcare outcomes management and planning will result in the improvement of overall health and well-being for individuals and the community-at-large.

ECONOMIC HEALTHCARE ANALYSIS

The economic evaluation of healthcare delivery has the potential to affect healthcare outcomes management and planning, which ultimately may affect the health and well-being of individuals and populations accessing healthcare services today. Economic evaluations of healthcare service delivery, if performed using rigorous scientific methodology, are among the most relevant research studies available to healthcare policy makers to aid in healthcare decision making.

When new healthcare interventions become available, issues as to whether investments should be made to adopt these interventions must be determined. Often, healthcare delivery systems make decisions to invest in new healthcare interventions based on minimizing the cost to the bottom line. This investment strategy ignores relevant outcomes data and information, leads to loss of productivity, and erodes healthcare constituency value (Brown et al., 2005).

Often, many healthcare interventions that cost more deliver more value for the dollar expended than interventions that are less costly. Healthcare delivery decision makers must look to gain the most value from those healthcare interventions for the healthcare resources expended, not to necessarily spend less money. The economic evaluation of healthcare interventions using cost-utility analysis incorporates all of the variables into appropriate and knowledgeable healthcare decision making.

Decisions to invest in cutting-edge technology and healthcare interventions often rely on analytical tools that compare financial returns on investment (ROI). These tools include the internal rate of return, economic value added, and net present value (NPV) analysis. Net present value analysis compares future financial returns on investment that are corrected for the time value of money to initial cash expenditure.

According to Brown et al. (2005), healthcare economic analysis is similar to NPV analysis for the following reasons:

- They involve cash investments in the form of capital expenditures (e.g., buildings, equipment, land, and other natural resources) and/or operational expenditures (e.g., human resources).
- They quantify benefits accrued measured in dollars for NPV analysis and healthcare outcomes management and planning in healthcare economic analysis.
- The principles of discounting and sensitivity analysis are included in both forms of analysis.
- Both forms of analysis involve a comparison of the benefits accrued to the financial investments in terms of an overall summary statistic.
- Both forms of analysis allow for multiple projects to be compared to one another.

It is important to note that when using any form of healthcare economic analysis, healthcare interventions that require a significant expenditure of capital dollars and are that will improve healthcare outcomes are the healthcare interventions that should be considered for analysis. Examples of healthcare interventions that meet the above criteria include a new drug delivery system based on computer-assisted physician order entry (CPOE), a genetic screening program, or the addition of a new medication to a managed care plan's formulary of drugs. The major criteria for any healthcare intervention considered for economic analysis is its proven clinical efficacy under controlled conditions and its effectiveness generalized to the population using evidence-based and value-based medicine principles and practices.

Healthcare economic evaluations may be broken down into four major categories for analysis: cost-minimization analysis, cost-benefit analysis, cost-effectiveness analysis, and cost-utility analysis. Each category of healthcare economic analysis provides different types of analysis on healthcare interventions being considered for implementation in a healthcare delivery system (Brown et al., 2005).

Cost-minimization analysis

Cost-minimization analysis compares two healthcare interventions of equal efficacy and effectiveness to determine which intervention is less costly (Brown et al., 2005). In this type of analysis, a critical assumption is made that the efficacy and effectiveness of the healthcare interventions being compared are equivalent. Given this assumption, the program with the lower cost is the preferred choice for widespread implementation in the healthcare delivery system. For example, a hypercholesterol drug equivalence trial demonstrates there is no difference in the efficacy and effectiveness between two new cholesterol-lowering drugs. Using cost-minimization analysis, the less costly of the two new drugs should be selected for the formulary as the preferred choice to be used at the point of care to maximize healthcare outcomes from a clinical and financial perspective.

The major problem with cost-minimization analysis is that two healthcare interventions are rarely exactly equivalent in efficacy and effectiveness. For example, in the above equivalence trial described the therapeutic efficacy and effectiveness of each drug in lowering cholesterol levels to maximize clinical outcomes may be similar, but the side effects, the severity and frequency of side effects, and the incidence of side effects associated with each drug will more than likely be different. Thus, this chosen form of healthcare economic analysis does not truly compare drugs with equivalent value.

Cost-benefit analysis

Cost-benefit analysis compares the costs expended on a healthcare intervention with the costs saved as a result of the healthcare intervention's implementation into the healthcare delivery system (Brown et al., 2005). Costs may be measured monetarily in dollars. However, for efficacy and effectiveness to be measured monetarily, healthcare outcomes must be converted into dollars. This type of healthcare economic analysis requires placing a monetary value on all healthcare outcomes pertinent to the analysis including length of life, quality of life, functionality, morbidity, and mortality. For example, if the healthcare outcome of interest in the analysis is length of life in years, the cost-benefit analysis may use an individual's annual earnings per life-year saved as the monetary measure of efficacy and effectiveness.

When other factors such as quality of life and potential complications from implementing the healthcare intervention must be considered, cost-benefit analysis will usually measure efficacy and effectiveness using a willingness-to-pay methodology. Using the willingness-to-pay methodology, individual patients studied in the analysis are asked how much money they would be willing to spend to completely avoid a particular negative healthcare outcome.

Cost-benefit analysis should report results in the form of a *net benefit* in dollars. This is the difference between the monetary values of the health benefits derived minus the cost of implementing the healthcare intervention. Assigning a price to a healthcare outcome is a difficult task and may only be possible in a limited number of situations. The main disadvantage in using cost-benefit analysis is that individual subjects studied in the analysis often come from distinctly different sociodemographic backgrounds. Therefore, their willingness to spend dollars to avoid a particular negative healthcare outcome can be vastly different based on annual income, educational level, and cultural influences. In addition, whether the individual subject studied has an appropriate amount of health insurance, or whether they are under- or uninsured may have a direct effect on their willingness to pay to avoid a negative healthcare outcome. It is obvious that the differences sociodemographically among individual subjects may be significant. Therefore, bias and confounding may be problematic when interpreting the data generated during the analysis.

Cost-benefit analysis without taking quality of life into account is more feasible. For example, the cost of a cochlear ear implant surgery for a deaf patient may be compared to the dollars saved by this patient being able to work and contribute to the gross national product (GNP) more effectively after surgery.

Cost-effectiveness Analysis

Cost-effectiveness analysis measures healthcare outcomes in terms of life-years gained, healthy years gained, asthma-free months gained, good-vision years gained, and so on, for the costs expended on implementing a particular healthcare intervention (Brown et al., 2005). The healthcare outcome for cost-effectiveness analysis is measured in units of effect gained for the healthcare resources expended. A common unit of effectiveness used in this form of healthcare economic analysis is length of life. Cost-effectiveness analysis frequently compares the cost per life-year saved between two potential healthcare outcomes.

Life-years saved is not an appropriate healthcare outcome measure if the healthcare intervention is designed to improve *quality* of life rather than *quantity* of life. In these instances, good-vision years gained, good-work years gained, disability-free years, or some other appropriate healthcare outcome may be used. Even then, cost-effectiveness analysis is not an all inclusive measure of quality of life parameters when compared to cost-utility analysis.

Regardless of the healthcare outcome unit chosen for this type of healthcare economic analysis, the purpose of a cost-effectiveness analysis is to compare the cost per healthcare outcome between the healthcare interventions under consideration. A study by Tengs et al. (1995) provides an excellent example of the different applications of cost-effectiveness analysis in the form of life-years saved. In this study, the 500 healthcare interventions were divided into three groups based on the following categories: medical interventions, injury reduction interventions, and environmental toxin control interventions.

Healthcare interventions included the treatment of contagious infectious diseases, the use of vaccinations, and the use of mammography for the detection of breast cancer. Injury reduction interventions included the adoption of flammability standards for children's sleepwear and clothing, setting highway speed limits, and random automobile inspections.

Environmental toxin control interventions included regulations governing acceptable lead levels in water, asbestos use, and radiation control standards. The mean or average cost to save one year of life in 2004 U.S. dollars per grouping of interventions was the following:

- A medical intervention cost an average of $24,298 dollars to save one year of life.
- An injury reduction intervention cost an average of $62,329 dollars to save one year of life.
- An environmental toxin control intervention cost an average of $3,623,000 dollars to save one year of life.

To further frame the importance of using cost-effectiveness analysis, at a cost of $81 million dollars, one life year could be saved by banning asbestos in automatic transmission components of automobiles whereas at a cost of $175 dollars, one life year could be saved instituting a comprehensive influenza immunization program (Torrence, Siegel, and Luce, 1996).

Cost-utility Analysis

Cost-utility analysis measures the value conferred by a healthcare intervention for the healthcare resources expended in dollars. The value conferred incorporates the improvement in both the quantity and quality of life. This value is measured in terms of the quality-adjusted life years gained (QALY gained) (Brown et al., 2005).

A utility is a measure of the strength of preference for a particular healthcare outcome and has conceptual foundation in healthcare economics and decision-based theory. The worth an individual places on that particular healthcare outcome is his/her individual utility. By using utilities, the quality of life associated with a particular healthcare outcome may have multiple critical indices that may be measured and reported with only one number after consolidation (usually in terms of a ratio as previously described).

Cost-utility analysis is the method of healthcare economic evaluation that allows for different healthcare outcomes of a healthcare intervention to be combined into one comprehensive, single measure of value. This type of healthcare economic analysis provides a more complete assessment of the efficacy and effectiveness of a healthcare intervention, but is not forced to assign monetary values in dollars to each healthcare outcome identified.

The healthcare outcome measure for cost-utility analysis is the healthcare resources expended in dollars per QALY gained. Measuring a healthcare outcome in terms of QALYs gained allows both morbidity and mortality to be combined into a single measure. Therefore, a cost-utility analysis may investigate the cost in dollars per QALY gained from the implementation of a particular healthcare intervention compared to any alternative healthcare intervention or no healthcare intervention.

Cost-utility analysis will allow for the construction of a value-based medicine quality standards database (Brown et al., 2005). Cost-utility analysis is the most comprehensive form of healthcare economic evaluation. The comprehensive nature of this analysis has the potential to combine all costs, benefits, and even adverse effects associated with any healthcare intervention into a final healthcare outcome of healthcare resources expended in dollars for the value gained in terms of those dollars spent per QALY.

THE FUTURE OF VALUE-BASED MEDICINE

Cost-utility analysis will become the instrument that allows for the creation of a comparable cost-utility database across all medical and surgical specialties of medicine (Brown et al., 2005).This specific type of healthcare economic analysis will serve as the foundation for a value-based medicine (VBM) quality standards database for all healthcare interventions and healthcare outcomes management and planning. Once a sufficient, valid, and reliable VBM database is developed, those healthcare interventions that are discovered to be harmful, of no benefit, or of negligible benefit on the basis of healthcare outcomes management and planning may be examined more closely to determine if it improves or should be eliminated from the healthcare delivery systems as a whole. As healthcare interventions are deemed to be more cost-utilitarian (described in the peer-reviewed medical literature as cost-effective), the allocation of healthcare resources may be funneled to fully implement these interventions into all healthcare delivery systems.

According to Brown et al. (2005), there are currently more than sufficient healthcare resources available in the U.S. healthcare delivery system to pay for healthcare interventions that provide value for all of the population. Value-based medicine provides the mechanism to conserve limited healthcare resources that can be appropriately allocated to provide healthcare interventions for all of the U.S. population regardless of economic status and the accessibility of insurance coverage. Value-based medicine will provide a standardized quality measurement that has been lacking in the U.S. healthcare delivery system for some time.

CHAPTER 11

Measuring Equity

INTRODUCTION TO MEDICAL ETHICS

The goals for the practice of medicine within any healthcare delivery system (especially in the United States) include the following:

- Promotion of health
- Prevention of disease
- Relief of pain and suffering
- Cure of disease
- Prevention of untimely death
- Improve functional status
- Education and counseling of patients
- To do no harm in the course of care

In promoting the goals of medical practice, clinicians face significant challenges biologically, psychologically, socially, environmentally, and technically. In managing these challenges, ethical issues arise that must be balanced with the goals of the practice of medicine.

There has been a transition in the U.S. healthcare delivery system that has taken a cottage-like healthcare industry and converted it to a large-scale institutional-like bureaucracy. The "cottage industry" medical practice flourished from the 1940s to the 1970s. It consisted of solo or small (two or three physicians) group medical practices that demanded face-to-face contact between clinician and patient at the point of care. Clinicians were paid on a fee-for-service basis. Any economic conflict-of-interest favored the clinician and there was an attitude of relative abundance with respect to allocation of healthcare resources.

There was little or no accountability for scientific rigor and the practice of medicine was based on the experience of the clinician and individual practice style. On the other hand, at the transition to managed care and the beginning of large scale institutional-like medical practice in the 1980s, the basic relationship between clinician and patient shifted to include a relationship between the institutions, managed care third-party administrators, and the patient. Evidence-based medicine, clinical practice guidelines, and accountability for scientific rigor with quality of care became the focus in medicine (and continues today). Any economic conflict-of-interest punishes the clinicians at the point of care and an attitude of relative scarcity with respect to allocation of healthcare resources exists.

The managed practice of medicine focuses on these main objectives that all healthcare facilities must quantify and report:

- Increase quality of clinical care
- Decrease cost of clinical care
- Increase access to healthcare delivery services
- Oversupply of healthcare delivery services
- Privilege of receiving clinical care
- Achieve greater economic efficiency
- Create conflicts of interests in how healthcare professionals are paid
- Regulation of clinical judgment, decision making, and clinical practice

This transition to managed clinical care within the U.S. healthcare delivery system has created ethical problems in the care of patients and the management of healthcare institutions.

To understand the basis for these ethical challenges, a short discussion on the basic principles of ethics is required. According to Beauchamp and Childress (1994), ethics is defined as the disciplined study of morality. Ethics assists people in understanding what their behavior ought to be towards others, what *virtues* ought to be cultivated in our character, and what *vices* ought to be avoided.

Preventive ethics is a subdiscipline of ethics that applies the principles and practices of ethics to in an effort to preempt the development of a critical event at the point of care. Preventive ethics is of great value in the delivery of healthcare services. Healthcare professionals and institutions act as the fiduciary of the patient. A healthcare fiduciary is someone who acts primarily to protect and promote the interests of the patient, blunts self-interest, and expects economic and other forms of self-interest to be fulfilled as the effect of taking good care of patients. In this system, patients agree to be cared for under the management strategies of managed practice at the point of care.

The ethical principles used in the process of preventive ethics within the healthcare delivery system interpret how clinical behavior can protect and promote the interests of the patient. The main principles of preventive ethics include beneficence (the clinicians' perspective), autonomy (the patients' perspective), and justice (Beauchamp and Childress, 1994).

The ethical principle of beneficence states that the healthcare professional's behavior in patient care provide greater good than harm to the patient from a rigorous clinical perspective. For example, greater good is the prevention of disease/premature death and harm is the pain and suffering without prevention of disease or death. The ethical principle of autonomy refers to the patient perception that the healthcare professional's behavior provides greater good than harm (e.g., informed consent). Justice refers to the clinician–patient relationship now affected by third parties that own or manage healthcare resources. Additionally, neither the clinician nor the patient have an overriding right to the use of privately and publicly owned healthcare resources. The ethical principle of justice manages disputes about the management of healthcare resources. In general, this principle requires individuals and institutions to render to each individual what is due to that individual. The response by the healthcare professional to the scarcity of resources at the bedside should be reasonable advocacy for meeting the patient's interests as determined in beneficence-based and autonomy-based clinical judgment. A more complete discussion of the ethical principle of justice follows these introductory comments on preventive ethics.

The first principle task of preventive ethics is to identify ethically justified forms of the economically disciplined healthcare fiduciary. This healthcare professional exhibits the cultivation of four character virtues: self-effacement, self-sacrifice, compassion, and integrity. The healthcare fiduciary is inherently motivated to protect and promote the patient's interest in an intellectually disciplined way.

What is the ethical challenge for the healthcare fiduciary today? Fiduciary obligations today must be subjected to economic discipline. What are the ethical obligations of patients in today's managed practice of medicine? Patients are obligated to take part in the informed consent process with their practitioners, avoid unreasonable care burdens with their families, and become prudent users of healthcare resources that the patient does not own. What are the ethical obligations of healthcare institutions in today's managed practice of medicine? Healthcare institutions are obligated to organize, deliver, or influence the delivery of healthcare as co-fiduciaries, to protect and promote the fiduciary responsibilities of the professionals who work in or for the institution, and to use healthcare resources only in ways for which ethical justification can be made.

The second principle task of preventive ethics in the managed practice of healthcare delivery is deciding how to fulfill the ethical obligation to provide patients the standard of care in healthcare services while both meeting other healthcare service missions and preserving fiscal viability for the healthcare institution and the healthcare delivery systems as a whole. The transition to the managed practice of medicine beginning in the 1980s resulted in third-party payers not tolerating the unmanaged practice of medicine (e.g., evidence-based medicine, clinical practice guidelines, disease management, preventive health care, etc.), freedoms lost by clinicians at the point of care (e.g., favorable economic conflict of interest and practicing without scientific discipline) and a standard of clinical and scientific-based medicine that is carefully and rigorously identified.

Sources of morality (Beauchamp and Childress, 1994) that shape the actions of all in the healthcare delivery system today include:

- Pluralistic society
- Rule of law (e.g., statutory, common, regulatory, and administrative)
- Historical experience
- Religious beliefs
- Professional education and training
- Individual and family experience

- Professional consensus
- Authorities and experience
- Institutional policies and practices

The basic tools of ethical decision making are those that include exhibiting intellectual criteria of clarity, consistency, coherence, applicability, and adequacy (Beauchamp and Childress, 1994). Each healthcare fiduciary must submit to the intellectual discipline required by such criteria. The healthcare fiduciary must engage in ethical analysis and develop clear concepts that can be used in arguments about what morality ought to be within the healthcare delivery system and in particular, when ethical issues arise at the point of care. An ethical argument is one that requires a coherent set of reasons that produce a conclusion as their logical consequence. Using the basic tools of ethical decision making assists the healthcare fiduciary in making an ethical argument.

The fundamental virtues of the healthcare fiduciary include directing the healthcare professional's attention primarily to the patient's interest and moving the healthcare professional to act to protect and promote the patient's interests (Beauchamp and Childress, 1994). These virtues are described below. Self-effacement is the willingness routinely to put aside differences that should not count in the care of patients (e.g., dress, speech, race, and gender). Self-sacrifice is the willingness to risk one's other relationships, as well as health, and even life threatened in and by the care of patients. Compassion is the willingness to acknowledge, to respond to, and to relieve the suffering and distress of others both intellectually (intuitive knowledge) and motivationally (action). Integrity is willingness to form rigorous, well-made clinical and ethical judgments about how to protect and promote the interest of others. Finally, legitimate self-interest has the requisites for providing good patient care, obligations owed to others outside of the healthcare profession and the healthcare delivery system, and individual activities beyond clinical practice of self-growth.

The expected ethical behavior of patients today needs to be defined as well. Patients have ethical obligations to their healthcare professionals to be serious partners in the informed consent process. They have ethical obligations to respect the autonomy of their healthcare professionals. Patients have ethical obligations to other patients, families, payers, institutions, and society not to impose long-term care burdens that are judged to be unreasonable. Patients' positive rights (e.g., claims on others for their resources or resources held in common in society) are justifiably limited when those rights place demands on scarce healthcare resources. Finally, patients have ethical obligations to institutions and society to be prudent savers for their own healthcare costs.

The morality of society within healthcare delivery also needs to be defined. Healthcare policy enacted by statute or regulation is at best temporary health care. Political consensus that enacted policy can be reliably expected regularly to collapse at unpredicted intervals. Society has a vested interest in preserving the fiduciary character of healthcare professions and institutions.

EQUITY AND JUSTICE

Equity is a principle that combines fairness, justice, and equality. There are different ways of deciding how healthcare delivery goods and services are to be distributed to individuals and populations in a fair, just, and equal manner. Ethical theories assist in this process of distribution of healthcare delivery goods and services (Sinclair, 2000).

Equity may be assessed by comparing levels of health and well-being. Equity may also be assessed by individuals' and populations' ability to obtain healthcare goods and services. There are two major forms of equity: horizontal and vertical equity. Horizontal equity involves allocating equal healthcare resources to patients with similar disease states as well as equal access to healthcare services for individuals and populations with equal needs. Vertical equity involves providing unequal treatment for unequal needs of individuals and populations. Vertical equity deliberately allocates healthcare resources in an unequal manner to those individuals and populations who are unequal in society. Vertical equity enables these individuals to overcome the effects of differences in society by allocating healthcare resources unequally. For example, diverting healthcare resources from healthier populations to populations with poorer health would be a form of vertical equity.

Horizontal equity requires the equal treatment of equals. This may involve equal healthcare resource allocation for people with equal needs based on population age, gender, and standardized mortality ratio. Additionally, it ensures that all equal patients wait the same length of time for treatment, and that the lengths of stay during treatment are also equal.

Horizontal equity may involve equal health status aimed at reducing inequalities in health status between populations.

Vertical equity involves unequal treatment for unequal needs. More healthcare resources are allocated to patients with serious diseases and health conditions than to those with less serious conditions. It may also involve financing health care according to the ability to pay. How does one decide what is fair, just, and equal in the delivery of healthcare services? There are principles that have been developed that assist and aid healthcare policy makers in these decisions and inform their implementation.

Equity and Ethical Theories

Equity is based on a number of ethical theories that describe how healthcare resources should be shared among the population. These ethical theories try to explain how people decide which acts are right and which acts are wrong. They are the basis for concepts of distributive justice and represent different views held about the relationship between the individual and society as a whole. Many of these ethical theories and concepts are universal and may be found in any culture. However, each theory has its advantages and disadvantages as well as alternative explanations of why people should strive for equity in healthcare delivery systems.

An ethical theory is a statement of principles that justify certain actions (Beauchamp and Childress, 1994). Ethical theories are sets of rules or guidelines which can be used to decide whether an act is right or wrong, whether the act is just and fair or unjust. Consequence-based ethical theories judge actions to be right or wrong according to the balance of their good or bad consequences. Thus, in any given situation, the right act is the act that produces the greatest net benefit to individuals within the population. Deontological ethical theories consider whether an action is right or wrong based on both the good or bad consequences of the action and individual motives that led to the person committing the action.

An example of a consequence-based ethical theory is Utilitarianism first described in the writings of Jeremy Bentham and John Stuart Mills. The essence of this ethical theory is that one should always act to produce the greatest net benefit or utility to individuals and welfare to society. Utilitarianism is the guiding ethical theory underlying modern economic theory. Utilitarian-based economists argue that there are utility-maximizing behaviors of individuals in a perfectly competitive market that will maximize economic efficiency and social welfare. In healthcare outcomes management and planning, Utilitarianism is the ethical basis for measuring quality-adjusted life years (QALY). Here the aim is to maximize the length and quality (however estimated) of life and to use the measure to decide how best to allocate healthcare resources fairly and justly.

Utilitarianism can be criticized along with other consequence-based ethical theories because it is only interested in producing the greatest net benefit to individuals in society through maximizing utility. As equity is not a primary concern, the approach could be used to justify inequalities. For example, a fair distribution of basic healthcare goods and services for everyone in a population could be seen as less necessary than another type of distribution considered to provide a greater overall benefit to society as a whole. Utilitarians are often criticized for their lack of concern regarding patient autonomy. The question of whose utility should be assessed in the construction of QALYs is often raised by critics of Utilitarianism. Is it justifiable to use community preferences to make healthcare decisions about individual cases or to use preferences of the well-off to prioritize services for the poor?

An example of a deontological ethical theory is Kantianism, first described by Immanuel Kant in the eighteenth century (Kant, 1985). Kant argued that morality is grounded in pure reason, not in tradition, conscience, or emotion. He also noted that an action is morally acceptable if and only if it is performed by an individual acting from a morally valid motive. Kant proposed that people should be guided in their actions by principles that could be accepted by all rational individuals as universal laws, which Kant called maxims. In a perfect world, all actions and choices would be guided by these maxims. Finally, Kant believed that individuals should choose to act from these generally acceptable motives. Kant called this moral autonomy.

John Rawls (1971) is best known for developing modern Kantianism on the themes of reason, equality, and autonomy. Rawls is in direct opposition to Utilitarianism in that he argues that individuals who live in a society must assist in improving the society for everyone. However, Rawls states that the rights of individuals cannot be legitimately sacrificed for the good of the community. He argues that one should act to improve the lives of the most disadvantaged. His argument suggests that the advantaged in society should plan and develop health services targeted towards the disadvantaged.

Kantianism fails to recognize that the rules of conduct should not be based solely on generalizability. However, ethical judgments, rules, and principles should be generalizable (Beauchamp and Childress, 1994). There may be occasions when maxims impose conflicting obligations, and this may lead to conflicts among individuals. As maxims are considered to be absolute, there is no way to determine which should take precedence. Situations may arise where it is impossible to choose which of a number of alternative acts is the most just.

Another ethical theory of justice is that of Rights theory or Liberal Individualism. Rights are justified claims that individuals and populations may make upon others or on society as a whole. These justified claims depend on the existence of a system of rules authorizing them. Moral rights are justified by moral principles and rules and one need not assert his/her individual rights in order to possess them (Sinclair, 2000).

Rights may be absolute *(prima facie)*, positive or negative. Many rights are correlated with obligations. Thus, the rights to receive something usually imply that there is an obligation on someone else, either a person or an institution, to provide it. Rights form the basis for Liberal Individualism, which aims to protect the freedom of the individual in society so that he/she may pursue his/her own individual ambitions (Beauchamp and Childress, 1994).

There are absolute rights that exist irrespective of circumstances. From a practical perspective, there are very few examples in society. In the United States, one is presumed innocent of an alleged illegal act unless proven guilty by due process in a court of law. *Prima facie* rights exist except where they conflict with an equal or overriding right. The right of healthcare workers to speak freely may conflict with the right of patient confidentiality. Positive rights require that one be provided with a particular healthcare good or service. For example, in the United States, hospitals are not allowed to refuse clinical care to anyone who is seeking legitimate healthcare services. Negative rights require that one be free from some action taken by others. There is usually a right to refuse medical treatment grounded in the principle of autonomy. This is also an example of a *prima facie* right as it can be overridden when individuals are considered to lack the capacity to make informed decisions. Ethical theories based on individual rights may be ideal for ensuring that everyone in society is equally entitled to a fair, just, and equal allocation of healthcare resources for legitimated healthcare needs.

Rights are based on a system of law used to enforce them. These rights are subject to the decisions of lawmakers. In an ideal democratic society, the lawmakers represent the will of the population because it is the individuals in the population that elect these lawmakers to represent their needs in society. In the real world, laws are often made by those with the personal power to enforce them. Rights are limited by the resources that are available. These rights may turn into paper rights when there are no resources to provide the level of healthcare goods and services that people are entitled to in society. In addition, a system that is based on the rights of individuals may give a disproportionate emphasis to serving individuals rather than the community-at-large. If decisions are made only on the basis of individual rights, irrespective of costs, resources could be wasted on a few costly cases rather than serving the good of the whole community-at-large.

Community-based theory, or communitarian theories, are ethical theories that place a greater emphasis on the values held by specific communities and includes their culture and traditions. Those that believe in ethical theory criticize liberal theories as lacking a real commitment to the general social welfare of the society as a whole. There are many different definitions of community, ranging from individual families to entire nations. Sinclair (2000) defines a community as a group of people who share a common set of understandings, practices, and language. Communitarianism is similar to Utilitarianism in that acts are judged according to the amount of good they do for the community. For example, some nations have "presumed consent laws" which permit the use of cadavaric organs for transplantation unless individuals have registered their dissent. These laws are justified in terms of the benefit to the community and society as a whole (Sinclair, 2000).

Communitarians believe in the need to develop living neighborhoods with their own particular identities and shared values. This concept is the basis for many public health initiatives. In addition, Communitarians tend to emphasize that local community practices and values should take priority over ethical theories when making moral decisions; a healthcare system based on such ideals would be responsive to local customs and culture. However, problems with this ethical theory may arise if a community believes, for example, that all children should be vaccinated because it is in the best interest of the community. This may present a moral and legal dilemma for those parents who dissent to childhood vaccination. Additionally, local communities may be at odds with their nation as a whole.

Common morality is the set of values shared by the members of a society which rise out of a common sense of tradition. Principle-based theories are founded on a number of principles of obligation that stem from the common morality of the society as a whole. They do not need to be grounded in pure reason or to be justified by any external agency within the society. The principles that are commonly considered to arise from the common morality are autonomy, beneficence, non-maleficence, and justice (Beauchamp and Childress, 1994). The respect for autonomy refers to the respect for individuals' decision making capacities and implies that all individuals are equally worthy of respect and dignity. Beneficence refers to how benefits are balanced against harms or costs to individuals. Non-maleficence refers to the issue of avoiding harm to individuals. Finally, justice refers to the distribution of benefits to individuals fairly and justly. These are *prima facie* principles. They have no inherent order of priority and they are subject to revision as necessary. These principles of common morality may be balanced against each other to form specific judgments. In fact, the same set of principles may actually justify decisions that actually contradict one another.

Principle-based, common-morality ethical theories comprise a set of guiding principles based on the values held by society as a whole and may be revised as necessary. These principles should command the support of the majority of individuals in the society as well as the healthcare delivery system functioning at all levels in the society: local, regional, and national. When there is a conflict among these principles, non-maleficence should take precedence above all of the others. Unfortunately, interpretation of these principles may be very subjective and requires general agreement as to what constitutes right and wrong in the society.

Equity and Need

Equity may be operationalized for the purpose of healthcare outcomes management and planning. Equity is directly related to personal healthcare needs and professional healthcare needs. Personal healthcare needs are individual perceptions of what a person believes he/she needs to become healthy, that he/she believes he/she has the means to pay for it and how much the individual is willing to pay for it. Professional healthcare needs are clinicians' perceptions of what they believe their patients need to become healthy. These needs can be measured as they relate to equity in two ways—one is access to healthcare goods and services, and the other way is to measure how much patients use the healthcare services. In addition, a step-wise process that allows for the appropriate selection of epidemiologic study design to measure equity exists.

Assessing whether a healthcare service is equitable may involve measuring and comparing structure, process, and outcomes (Donabedian, 2003). Structure designates the conditions under which health care is delivered. The conditions included may be *material resources,* such as facilities and equipment; *human resources* and *intellectual capital,* such as the number, variety, and qualifications of professional and support personnel; and *organizational characteristics* such as the medical and nursing staffs of a hospital or health system, kinds of management including supervision and performance review, and administrative functions including billing, accounts receivable, etc.

Process designates the activities that constitute the delivery of health care itself. This follows the continuum of care to include preventive care, acute care, chronic care, rehabilitative care, palliative care, and supportive care. The care is provided by clinicians and support personnel in a variety of settings including inpatient, outpatient, rehabilitative, and supportive centers of care. Families, friends, and the patients themselves are providers of health care as well.

Outcomes denote the changes in individuals and populations that can be attributed to healthcare delivery. Outcomes include changes in health status, changes in behavior or knowledge acquired by patients, family, and friends that may influence future delivery of health care, and the satisfaction of patients, family, and friends with the health care received and its outcomes. Structure, process, and outcomes may be compared between groups. To assess whether the differences found are inequitable, one must relate the difference to need.

The need for healthcare goods and services vary due to geographic factors, socioeconomic factors, ethnic factors, age, and gender. Geographical factors refer to the differences in prevalence and incidence of many diseases between different countries or regions. Socioeconomic factors refer to the association between deprivation, low standards of living, and poorer health status. Ethnic factors refer to the association between ethnicity and health such as Caucasians and cystic fibrosis or Africans and sickle cell disease. Age refers to the issues of being elderly and having a higher incidence and prevalence of chronic disease states such as coronary artery disease and cancers. Gender refers to the differences between males and females with gender-specific diseases like cervical and uterine cancer for females and prostate cancer for males.

A number of variables can assess a community or population's need for healthcare goods and services. Assessing the age and gender of the population and determining the standardized mortality ratio can provide useful outcomes measures for comparing the relative needs for healthcare goods and services of different communities and populations.

An observational study to measure equity, such as a cohort study or an ecological study, would best assess the community's need. There are two main processes by which one might analyze differences between communities with respects to equity and need: stratification and comparison. The stratification process involves separating groups into levels of need and analyzing differences in structure, process, and outcomes for each level of need. The comparison process involves comparing the study population with a reference population and comparing rates of use of healthcare goods and services with local, regional, national, or global rates. Even with these two processes, one must choose the definition of equity, either horizontal or vertical equity, to apply. The key to the analysis is to know what exactly to measure.

Mooney (1983) provides some insight into the operationalization of these concepts by identifying seven definitions of equality in healthcare delivery: equality of expenditure per capita, equality of structure per capita, equality of structure for equal need, equality of access for equal need, equality of utilization for equal need, equality of marginal met need, and equality of health.

Equality of expenditure per capita involves allocating the same amount of healthcare resources to every individual in the population. It makes no distinction between individuals in terms of their need for healthcare goods and services. It also does not consider the differences in the amount or quality of healthcare services that may be purchased by or for each individual.

Equality of structure per capita refers to allocating equal services to each individual, thus avoiding inequity due to variation in the cost of clinical care between points of care. There is no distinction between individuals in terms of their need for healthcare goods and services.

Equality of structure for equal need uses indicators of health needs based on age and gender to determine those sections of the population with greater requirements for healthcare goods and services. Extra healthcare resources are allocated to those groups within the population with greater measured need for healthcare goods and services. Determining a formula to qualify the differences in need between the groups remains an issue. This definition is an example of horizontal equity.

Equality of access for equal need involves assessing the costs patients incur to access the healthcare delivery system and trying to relate these to the need for healthcare goods and services. To improve the quality of care, more healthcare resources are allocated to those groups within the population who incur the greatest individual cost in obtaining healthcare goods and services. This group often represents groups in rural and health physician shortage areas who must travel to access adequate healthcare delivery. This is an example of vertical equity.

Equality of utilization for equal need allows for different patterns of healthcare utilization within different groups of the population. Often those groups, which are more deprived, make the least use of the available healthcare delivery goods and services. This definition of equity proposes an even greater allocation of healthcare resources to be used by the most deprived communities until they are using healthcare goods and services at the same rates as other deprived groups within the population. This is another example of vertical equity.

Equality of marginal met need accepts that differences exist in the costs of meeting healthcare delivery needs in different communities. It would only be possible to achieve an equitable allocation of healthcare resources to each community in whatever amounts are necessary for them all to provide the same healthcare delivery goods and services rank ordered by each group.

Finally, equality of health refers to the assumption that it is not sufficient to provide fewer allocations of healthcare resources to the more deprived groups within the population but that these groups should receive a disproportionately greater allocation of healthcare resources in order to achieve the same healthcare status and outcomes as more affluent groups. This is the best example of vertical equity.

Equality of access is about equality of opportunity to receive an adequate amount of healthcare goods and services to meet both personal and professional needs. Access to healthcare delivery services does not consider whether individuals or populations actually take advantage of such opportunities. Each individual and the population as a whole must be made aware that healthcare resources are available for access and they might benefit from them.

Equality of utilization requires that those with the greatest personal need for healthcare resources perceive that they have this need. These individuals must have adequate and easy access to healthcare delivery services so they may take advantage of the healthcare goods and services offered.

Assessing Equity: A Practical Approach

The process of assessing equity is difficult at best. First, there are multiple definitions of equity to choose from. Second, issues of maintaining efficacy, effectiveness, and efficiency while ensuring equity may result in a trade-off. For example, it may be costly to have an equal distribution of healthcare facilities for the treatment of rare diseases. In addition, smaller numbers of patients per facility may also affect effectiveness as a minimal number of operations may be required to maintain the performance of the healthcare intervention (Mooney, 1983).

The first step in the process of assessing equity is to choose the appropriate definition of equity. Then, one can determine the point to measure, such as whether to assess equity in terms of access or utilization. Access is very difficult to measure. A straightforward way to measure access is to examine the time or distances patients must go to receive healthcare services. One would need to consider that those who can afford transportation will have greater access to healthcare delivery in general. Those patients with children, the elderly, or the disabled will have less access. Additionally, one might want to consider waiting times at the point of care, user charges (patient co-pays) at the point of care, or availability of information about the healthcare delivery goods and services that are available to patients at the point of care of choice.

Utilization of healthcare delivery services is much easier to measure (Sinclair, 2000). Routine data and information are collected on a variety of healthcare services including, but not limited to, surgical procedures, prescriptions, and immunizations. In addition, the sociodemographic backgrounds, age, gender, and employment of patients are collected today. If routine data and information are not easily available, special surveys at the point of care may be initiated to collect utilization data about a particular population of patients. Of course, this could become very costly but the survey could be very specific in the utilization data and information one wishes to collect and analyze.

The next step is to consider the population who will be served by the healthcare interventions being evaluated. This population of interest is likely to include communities comprised of people of different ages, gender, ethnicity, and socioeconomic class.

The third step is to assess equity in terms of need, both personal and professional. If the healthcare intervention under consideration is a surgical procedure (e.g., coronary artery bypass), then one may wish to assess the rates of coronary artery disease that require this procedure. If the healthcare intervention under consideration is a clinical preventive service, then one may wish to assess the rates of the events that one is seeking to prevent (e.g., prostate cancer, breast cancer, and hypercholesterolemia).

The next step is to relate either access or utilization to personal and professional need. For example, when considering coronary artery disease health promotion, one may assess need by using surveys of the prevalence of risk factors like smoking or hypertension by social class, gender, age, etc. One might consider assessing utilization by the number of patients receiving health promotion information at the point of care.

Finally, in addition to studying the relationship between access and utilization of healthcare delivery services and personal and professional need, one may wish to evaluate healthcare services' availability to those of equal need irrespective of age, gender, ethnicity, and socioeconomic status.

CONCLUSION

Ethical challenges face clinicians today as they prepare to make decisions regarding the allocation of limited healthcare resources. In an attempt to anticipate these ethical challenges, preventive ethics has emerged as the discipline used by clinicians to assist in making healthcare decisions based on accepted ethical principles.

Healthcare outcomes may be directly affected by the ethical dilemmas that clinicians must deal with as they make decisions about who will get what healthcare resources, when, where, and how. Acting within accepted norms of morality, the decision making process is guided so that the patient always remains central to the process, guaranteeing equitable distribution of healthcare resources and maximizing positive healthcare outcomes.

CHAPTER 12

Population-based Medicine in Healthcare Outcomes Management and Planning

THE POINT OF CARE

Doing the *right* thing,
In the *right* amount,
In the *right* way,
At the *right* time.

The battleground for all of healthcare delivery today is at the point of care for the patient. From the hospital bed to the emergency room stretcher to the clinician's examination table to the patient's own bed, the point of care is the focus for healthcare services. Several issues arise when considering what healthcare services are best suited for the patient, a medical practice, or a community-at-large. What is the right thing to do for the patient (i.e., ethical and cultural considerations)? What are the right reasons for providing the healthcare services (i.e., ethical, cultural, quality, and outcomes considerations)? How much should and may be done for the patient (i.e., ethical, economic, quality, and outcomes considerations)? When should care be given (i.e., cultural considerations and the continuum of care)? Finally, where should care be delivered (i.e., continuum of care)?

According to Leon R. Kass, MD (1985), American medicine at the end of the 20th century was not well. He noted that the cost of medical care was on the rise and not easily and equitably accessible to all. Clinicians were being asked to see too many patients leading to an increase in medical errors, failures to diagnose, functional impairment, and inadequate therapeutics. A growth in both professional and patient power was on the rise in the face of significant federal, state, and local regulatory and statutory changes; thus the healthcare delivery system was a bureaucracy growing faster than the federal government. Kass states, "Medicine, as well as the community that supports it, appears to be perplexed regarding its purpose." Kass described his goals of medicine as the following: the healthy human being, indulgence or gratification aiming at pleasing the patient's desires and wishes (i.e., demand management), social and behavioral adjustment leading to changes in morality and society, the alteration of human nature, and the prolongation of human life.

Kass (1985) declares that:

> health appears to be a matter of more and less, a matter of degree, and standards of health seem to be relative to persons, and also relative to time of life in each person . . . health is a natural standard or norm-not a moral norm, not a 'value' as opposed to a 'fact', not an obligation-a state of being reveals itself in activity as a standard of bodily excellence or fitness, relative to each species and to some extent to individuals, recognizable if not definable and to some extent attainable...health is the well-working of the organism as a whole, an activity of the living body in accordance with its specific excellences.

Much of what Dr. Kass stated in the 1980s applies to the issues of healthcare delivery today. The use of outcomes management and planning helps to define health and well-being for the patient, for a population, and for a community. It provides a roadmap for knowing, "what is the right action to perform at the point of care" (Roadmaps, 2002). The American Medical Association (AMA) in partnership with the U.S. Department of Health and Human Services (DHHS) developed a program for health professionals called, "Roadmaps for Clinical Practice" (Roadmaps, 2002). The program aimed to help clinicians identify and use strategies to reduce disparities in health outcomes through integrating disease prevention and health promotion into routine medical care at the point of care. This program was established out of a need to address changes in the health status of the American population; the U.S. population is becoming older and more diverse; preventive and chronic care is increasingly joining curative and acute primary care; chronic disease management is becoming more prominent in many medical practices; more patients want active involvement in their health care; financial mechanisms supporting health care are changing; emphasis is increasingly placed on healthcare concerns of access, cost, quality, and outcome.

The above changes have had a significant impact on how health and healthcare delivery are perceived in the United States. Chronic disease states are becoming multifactorial in their etiology (i.e., genetic, environmental, or a combination of both) and are best treated with a multifaceted approach throughout the continuum of care. A shift in the way healthcare services are provided with an emphasis on disease prevention and health promotion is required to ameliorate many of the chronic diseases and their associated risk factors. A population-based approach at the point of care addressing the individual patient, a medical practice, or a community-at-large is one of many ways to address chronic disease management. Addressing factors that lead to chronic disease in the individual patient or the community-at-large will lead to a healthier and more functional population. Population-based medicine provides strategies to integrate clinical and public health prevention efforts at the point of care.

A systematic national effort to index and track the health status of the U.S. population is exemplified by the Public Health Service's *Healthy People* initiative. *Healthy People* 2010 (HP 2010) initiative is the third decade-spanning iteration of key health objectives for the United States. The goals of HP 2010 are to increase the quality of and years of healthy life for all Americans by eliminating health disparities including the differences in rates of mortality, morbidity, incidence, prevalence, burden of disease, and other adverse health conditions among specific population groups in the United States. A list of ten leading health indicators (LHIs) was also established in HP 2010 to provide a "snapshot" of health status and to permit clinical and public health professionals to better target health promotion and disease prevention interventions (see Table 12-1). In addition, the LHIs allow for the tracking of health status in individual patients, a medical practice, and the community-at-large. The indicators chosen extend beyond the health characteristics of individuals or populations to include social, environmental, and healthcare delivery system factors that affect health, such as violence, air pollutants, and access to care. Achieving the goals and leading health indicators of "Healthy People 2010" relies on available research that suggests a comprehensive, simultaneous, and coordinated effort involving disease prevention and health promotion across the continuum of care be established at all the points of care. By using these three roles of action: provision of direct preventive services, management and organization of preventive health services at the point of care, and advocacy within clinical settings, communities, and organized medicine, all health professionals can choose a venue for contribution to an improve the overall quality of life for all Americans today and in the future.

The health of the patient at the point of care can be addressed at the level of the individual patient and also at the level of a well-defined population (American Medical Association, 2002). Factors within the patient's community-at-large should be considered if they contribute to an individual patient's health and well-being. The patient's community may be an excellent resource of healthcare delivery services for physicians at the point of care to impact positively on the outcomes management of their patients. Population-based medicine provides strategies to integrate clinical and community prevention efforts at the point of care to improve clinical performance, financial performance, patient satisfaction, and quality of life for patients in a medical practice or community level.

Table 12-1   Healthy People 2010 Leading Health Indicators

1. Promote daily physical activity.
2. Promote good nutrition and healthier weights.
3. Prevent and reduce tobacco use.
4. Prevent and reduce substance abuse.
5. Promote responsible sexual behavior including abstinence.
6. Promote mental health and well-being.
7. Promote safety and reduce violence.
8. Promote healthy environments.
9. Prevent infectious disease through immunization.
10. Increase access to quality health care.

Table created from material in Roadmaps for clinical practice: a primer on population-based medicine. Chicago, IL: American Medical Association, 2002. pg. 1–3.

Population-based medicine, according to Lipkin and Lybrand (1982), has various approaches to medical care for groups based on common sociodemographic characteristics, risk factors, or diseases. This approach involves characterizing a population, identifying the healthcare problems of greatest priority, delivering healthcare services, and adapting clinical and administrative procedures at the point of care that are responsive to the identified health problems, and assessing health outcomes and providing feedback to the patients. The promise of population-based medicine depends on the following five points (American Medical Association, 2002):

- Meeting the needs of individual patients by concentrating on groups of patients
- Understanding where to direct limited healthcare resources
- Meeting evidence-based preventive guideline recommendations
- Developing systems at the point of care to effectively involve all deliverers of healthcare services in meeting the needs of patients
- Developing a comprehensive outcomes management program using available data to get the most "bang for the buck" in providing healthcare delivery services for patients and managing the point of care

The biopsychosocial model of healthcare delivery serves as the framework for population-based medicine. The one-to-many physician-group relationships consist of identifying a denominator population and addressing the chosen populations biopsychosocial health needs in a systematic manner. Classic continuous quality improvement using the "plan-do-check-act" approach is very well suited to applying a systematic process to healthcare delivery services. It removes the possibility of wide variations in the collection, storage, retrieval, and reporting of data. The denominator population can be classified into three levels (American Medical Association, 2002):

- Active patient population at the point of care within the last calendar year.
- Point of care community including members of the patient's household.
- Members of the community-at-large that are within the service area of the point of care but not necessarily receiving healthcare services at that specific point of care.

Population-based medicine uses a multitude of approaches including health promotion screening activities (e.g., age-appropriate cancer screening), comprehensive preventive health services for high-risk populations (e.g., adolescents, elderly), and comprehensive chronic disease programs (e.g., diabetes, congestive heart failure, asthma). Population-based medicine has two major components: a population healthcare delivery perspective and systematic opportunities for health promotion and disease prevention at the point of care.

POPULATION HEALTH PERSPECTIVE

Abraham Flexner wrote the following in 1910:

> His (the physician's) relationship was formerly to his patient—at most to his patient's family; and it was almost altogether remedial. If the patient had something the matter with him; the doctor was called in to cure it. Payment of the fee ended the transaction. But the physician's function is fast becoming social and preventive, rather than individual and curative. Upon him society relies to ascertain, and through measures essentially educational to enforce, the conditions that prevent disease and make positively for physical and moral well-being.

Advances in medical technologies, vaccines, and pharmaceuticals, along with the separation of medical and public healthcare delivery diverted the attention of physicians' medical education on the social and preventive roles envisioned by Flexner in 1910 (American Medical Association, 2002). The biomedical approach, which searches for causes of disease and their direct effects along with disparities in health status and health outcomes have become a major concern at the point of care and all levels of government. Population-based medicine requires strategies to:

- Reduce the personal need for health care through health promotion and disease prevention for individuals and communities-at-large
- Reduce the inappropriate demand for healthcare delivery services through health education and shared-decision making for patients
- Reduce the inappropriate underuse and overuse of healthcare delivery services through efficient statutory, regulatory, and administrative policies and procedures along with better patient-physician communication
- Increase the delivery of appropriate healthcare services through the use of evidence-based medicine, clinical practice guidelines, contin-

uous quality improvement, and outcomes management amongst all the constituencies of healthcare delivery.

A population health perspective is a "view of care that places the patient as central while recognizing that the patient exists in a specified context with geopolitical boundaries as well as sociocultural definition, each of which creates major effects on care" (Lipkin, 1982). A population health perspective recognizes interdependency of health and societal factors such as environment, socioeconomic status, physical, emotional, and social functioning, and lifestyle on patients, populations of patients, and communities-at-large (Harper, 1994). Achieving these outcomes requires the adherence to a continuum of preventive interventions applied to both individuals and communities-at-large. The American Association of Medical Colleges (1998) asserts that physicians should have the ability to "assess the health needs of a specific population; implement and evaluate interventions to improve the health of that population; and provide care for individual patients in the context of the culture, health status and health needs of the populations of which that patient is a member."

There are several principles that promote a population health perspective (Harper, 1994). Incorporating these principles into medical care can help to optimize health in the following manner:

- Provide a holistic view to treat patient's unique characteristics and also the societal influences on the patient
- Use a systems approach to coordinate and integrate the delivery of care by using multidisciplinary teams and multiorganizational arrangements for referral
- Follow an epidemiological foundation to improve objectivity in clinical and policy decision making
- Use an anthropologic view to understand the patient's perspective of his/her health
- Use distributive justice to recognize and reduce the unequal distributions of illness, disease, disability, and death across different groups.

The ability to apply population health perspective principles to population-based medicine to achieve socially responsible clinical and financial outcomes for individuals and the communities-at-large requires the healthcare delivery system to rely on clinical acumen, teamwork, and the power of advocacy for community change. The major goal of this endeavor would be to identify groups of patients on which to focus a concentrated set of preventive interventions and integrate individual diagnostic and management strategies in the context of family, cultural, and community factors. Additional goals would include ensuring access to high quality, cost-efficient healthcare delivery services for all people and promoting effective community programs for populations of people with specific healthcare needs.

DISEASE PREVENTION AND HEALTH PROMOTION

There are two basic reasons for concentrating on integrating disease prevention and health promotion into the clinical practice of healthcare delivery services (American Medical Association, 2002): the burden of disease caused by personal and preventable behaviors and the effectiveness of clinical preventive interventions. The use of tobacco, poor dietary habits, lack of exercise, substance abuse, and irresponsible sexual behavior are personal behaviors that were responsible for over half of all deaths in 1990. By 1999, heart disease and cancer were leading the list of causes of death despite considerable efforts at education. Thus, the mortality rate for several conditions that have a personal behavior component to their etiology decreased.

Although the data that is available on the contribution of health risk behaviors to disease and premature mortality clearly demonstrates a cause-and-effect relationship, many people continue to engage in these detrimental personal health practices. A study examining the rate of healthy behaviors occurring in the state of Michigan (Centers for Disease Control and Prevention, 2001) found that only three percent of all respondents reported engaging in four healthy practices: not smoking, maintaining a normal weight, regular exercise, and eating a healthy diet. The death rates and the cost to society as a whole are high as a result of unhealthy personal health practices. Morbidity and mortality resulting from unhealthy personal health practices can be reduced through early intervention in disease history or before the disease even develops (Van Gaal, 1997; Williamson, 1997; Oster, 1999; Higgins, 1993; Petty, 1993; Demers, 1990; Wee, 1999).

Healthcare providers recognize the value of providing clinical preventive services. Improved healthy lifestyles, decreased physical, psychological, and social impairment, and extended life expectancy with high functionality and quality of life are all recognized outcomes of disease prevention and health promotion.

Unfortunately, the benefits of clinical and community preventive interventions are overshadowed by the many barriers to implement critical healthcare delivery services. The lack of reimbursement by third-party payers has caused providers to place a less high priority on the supply of clinical preventive services. The fact that providers must see more patients for more acute and chronic diseases at the point of care to generate higher revenues, has also resulted in less office visit time to perform preventive care and health counseling. There has not been a coordinated effort (both privately and publicly) to provide evidence-based clinical guidelines to assist providers in deciding which screening services will provide the most sensitivity and specificity for the early detection of disease. Uncertainty amongst clinicians regarding the effectiveness of preventive interventions and the relative effectiveness of offering different preventive services has created a tension regarding causing unnecessary harm among healthy individuals. Finally, the lack of a well-designed and developed healthcare delivery system in the United States has resulted in fragmented healthcare delivery services and a failure to commit to the continuum of care at the points of care. Because patients are not effectively and efficiently cared for through a coordinated effort administratively and electronically, healthcare services are duplicated and open to failure to follow up on pertinent positive clinical testing.

Prevention is traditionally broken into three levels: primary, secondary, and tertiary clinical preventive services. Primary prevention treats disease-free individuals to prevent the onset of a particular condition or disease. An example of a primary preventive service is the routine age-appropriate immunization of children and adults. Secondary prevention treats individuals with a preclinical disease, or risk factors for that disease, to prevent the clinical expression of the disease. For example, Pap smears are performed to detect metaplastic and dysplastic changes in the cells of the cervix before the development of full-blown cervical cancer. Obviously the clinical outcomes will be different for an individual who has precancerous changes compared to an individual with cancer. Tertiary prevention treats individuals with a clinical disease to prevent further impact from the disease. For example, a diabetic patient will be encouraged to eat a healthy diet, get appropriate exercise, and follow a medication regime to prevent complications from the progression of poorly treated diabetes.

Another classification (Froom, 2000) outlines the target population at each level of prevention and identifies objectives that can be developed into an action plan to improve clinical outcomes for the patient. Primary prevention targets individuals without a specific medical condition and reduces their exposure to etiologic agents of disease (i.e., isolation), assists in developing individual resistance to disease (i.e., lifestyle modification), screens for and treats risk factors of disease in asymptomatic patients with a view to their reduction (i.e., adolescent sexual behavior), and promotes individual and population resistance to a causative agent (i.e., immunization and chemoprophylaxis). Secondary prevention targets individuals with medical conditions who are asymptomatic and screens these individuals for asymptomatic disease with view of early treatment (i.e., diabetes). Tertiary prevention targets individuals with symptomatic medical conditions and tries to prevent recurrence of the medical condition (i.e., hyperlipidemia treatment), prevents complications from the medical condition (i.e., medication regimen in treating diabetes), provides treatment of acutely symptomatic patients with view of cure, palliation, or reduction of mortality (i.e., antibiotics treating bacterial infections), and rehabilitation when the medical condition results in physical, psychological, or social impairment (i.e., physical or occupation therapy).

There are three dimensions (American Medical Association, 2002) of a disease process important to those clinicians engaging in providing clinical preventive services. The disease state dimension consists of two stages, "disease" or "no disease." Disease onset is when the "no disease" state becomes a "disease" state. The second dimension, symptom status, is when an individual has a disease and they are either asymptomatic or symptomatic. When a patient with a disease begins to develop symptoms, disease detection begins. The third and final dimension has to do with prevention activities, including assessment. Assessment includes gathering of information through clinical interview, anthropomorphic measurements, or standardized instruments. Screening is done with the hope of detecting risk behavior or disease earlier than the behavior or disease would ordinarily be detected after onset.

Health promotion is an integral component of disease prevention. Health promotion refers to a variety of strategies for improving conditions associated with achieving a healthy lifestyle such as adequate physical activity and eating a healthy diet. Health promotion can be delivered at the individual, population, and community-at-large levels. It is a key component of primary prevention and uses a host of techniques to help individuals achieve health and well-being.

There are well recognized barriers to providing clinical preventive services at the point of care (Frame, 1992). The barriers are divided into three categories: the healthcare delivery system, the physician, and the patient. The healthcare delivery system's barriers include issues related to inadequate payer reimbursement or employer support, lack of health insurance coverage, population mobility, lack of a primary care clinician to coordinate screening, and sporadic screening programs that are evidence-based and age appropriate. The physician's barriers to clinical preventive services include uncertainty about recommendations and the value of clinical preventive screening tests, poor administrative organization at the point of care, inadequate allotment of time for screening, and delayed gratification waiting to see positive, healthy behavior as a result of screening. The patient's barriers include a lack of knowledge about the benefits of screening, the costs of screening, physical and psychological effects associated with selected screening examinations along with false positive findings, and an overall unwillingness to pursue a healthy lifestyle. However, in the past decade, a growing body of peer-reviewed literature has demonstrated that a systematic team approach at the point of care toward clinical preventive services can improve clinical, financial, and satisfaction outcomes as well as overcome the barriers outlined by Frame (Woodruff, Carney, and Dietrich, 1992).

An effective systems approach to clinical preventive service at the point of care consists of tools, established routines, and shared responsibility among clinicians, staff, and the patients. A model was developed through a project supported by the National Cancer Institute called the *Cancer Prevention in Community Practice Project* (Woodruff, Carney, and Dietrich, 1992). The functions of this model system are fourfold:

1. Identifying a patient's need for evidence-based age-related clinical preventive services.
2. Monitoring the patient's age-related preventive health needs over time to insure clinical services are provided at regular intervals.

3. Reinforcing positive healthy behavior as an outcome of screening programs.
4. Obtaining feedback on the percentage of patients receiving age-related clinical preventive services to monitor outcomes management.

This model system is similar to the principles of continuous quality improvement (i.e., "plan-do-check-act"). Goals for the design and implementation of this model for providing clinical preventive services at the point of care must be set in accordance with objectives outlined by evidence-based peer-reviewed literature. This approach is also implemented incrementally to allow for proper evaluation and changes that enhance the outcomes of screening programs at the point of care.

HEALTH RISK ASSESSMENT

Before initiating a preventive clinical intervention, the importance of the target condition or risk factor must be assessed. A target condition is defined (Dever, 1997) as the disease or health outcome that the preventive clinical intervention avoids (primary prevention), identifies early (secondary prevention), or prevents from occurring (tertiary prevention). The relative importance of a target condition can be assessed by its frequency and severity. Frequency is measured by incidence rate (i.e., the number of new cases of a target condition during the given time period in a defined population at risk for developing the target condition) and prevalence rates (i.e., the total number of new and old cases of a given target condition during the given time period in a defined population at risk for developing the target condition). Severity can be measured in terms of morbidity, mortality, survival rates, cost, and quality of life. Populations that exhibit higher frequencies or greater severity of target conditions are good candidates for preventive clinical interventions.

Risk factors are defined as characteristics that are either directly related to or more likely to lead to the target condition(s). Risk factors may include demographic qualities (e.g., age, gender, ethnicity, income, education), behaviors (e.g., smoking, inappropriate sexual activity, unhealthy eating habits, alcohol intake and driving), environmental factors (e.g., occupation, geographic location, sanitation, living conditions), and healthcare system factors (e.g., access to care, preferences for healthcare services). The relative importance of risk factors can be determined by their frequency and magnitude in the target population. The magnitude of an association between a risk factor and a target condition can be calculated as measures of risk (American Medical Association, 2002). Each measure of risk has separate and distinct implications for disease prevention and the application of preventive clinical interventions at the point of care.

Relative risk measures the association between exposure to a particular risk factor (smoking) and a disease (lung cancer). Relative risk is reported as a ratio of exposure to disease. It shows how a change in the amount of exposure leads to a change in amount of disease. It is often applied at the individual or patient level. Attributable risk shows the potential for disease prevention (or risk factor modification) in a population if the exposure is eliminated. Attributable risk is the proportion of disease or risk attributed to a specific exposure. An example of modifying attributable risk in a population might be the following: among those in the population who smoke, how much lung cancer would be prevented if they stopped smoking?

Identifying target conditions and risk factors in an individual or population can lead to successful preventive clinical interventions. However, incremental success is the key to making long-standing changes for healthy lifestyles. For example, it is better to make small, incremental changes in a large number of people than to make large, global changes in small number of people.

According to Altman (1995),

> A population approach is considered a viable strategy for disease prevention because societal benefit that accrues from large numbers of people lowering their risk a small amount often exceeds the benefits obtained from larger risk changes among the smaller number of people at highest risk.

Therefore, preventive clinical interventions that demonstrate minor effectiveness in terms of relative risk may have significant impact on the population in terms of attributable risk if the target condition is common and associated with significant morbidity and mortality.

Highly effective preventive clinical interventions in terms of relative risk that are applied to a small high-risk group may save fewer lives than a preventive clinical intervention with less clinical effectiveness that is applied to large numbers of people at risk. For example, if the reduction in mortality with a specific preventive clinical intervention is 50 percent and the deaths per year from the target condition is ten, then five deaths are prevented with the specific preventive clinical intervention. On the other hand, if the reduction in mortality with a specific preventive clinical intervention is one percent and the deaths per year from the target condition is 100,000, then the specific preventive clinical intervention prevented 1000 total deaths.

Clinicians are accustomed to using the biomedical model approach and applying medical interventions that change the health status of most individuals they treat. Population-based medicine requires clinicians to value preventive clinical interventions applied to many patients in hopes of obtaining successful clinical outcomes with a small number and disease prevention as much as disease cured. At the point of care, clinicians are often able to modify preventive clinical interventions to patient risks. For example, at the point of care a clinician determines which patients are smokers and then intervenes in specific ways with these patients to provide preventive clinical interventions geared to patients with low health literacy. General public health campaigns would then serve to reinforce the efforts of the clinicians at the point of care. The main advantage of using preventive clinical interventions at the point of care is that *all* patients in a practice site are available for the clinician to guide into the intervention in hopes of increasing the number of patients with a successful outcome as a direct result of the intervention.

Assessing risk factors in a population at the point of care is an everyday activity. How risk factors are perceived and the attempts to measure risk factors are bound by cultural influences. Everyone has the propensity to take risks. This propensity varies from individual to individual within a population. This propensity is influenced by the potential rewards of risk taking. Perceptions of risk are influenced by experience of accident losses (one's own and others). Individual risk-taking decisions represent a balancing act in which perceptions of risk are weighed against propensity to take risk. Accident losses are, by definition, a consequence of taking risks; the more risks an individual takes, the greater both the rewards and losses he or she incurs will be. The risk-taking actions of others, along with individual behavior, can directly affect the outcomes noted from both healthy and unhealthy activities.

There are significant uncertainties and limitations in the data gathered when trying to understand the healthcare outcomes from risk activities.

However, information gathered can be used to make shared decisions about patient's health activities and control measures based on individual risks and the potential population disease burden. Political, social, and economic factors influence risk characterization. This leads to the development of the scientific discipline of health risk management. Health risk management is defined as the principles, criteria, or prevailing techniques used to identify, investigate, analyze, evaluate, and select the most advantageous methods reducing, modifying, correcting, or eliminating identifiable risks. Health risk management is useful to control the use of limited healthcare resources in the face of unlimited healthcare wants by consumers. It is the demand side of the health economics equation that is the next area of concentration in population-based medicine.

Americans have become increasingly aware that lifestyle choices can have significant consequences for their health and well-being (Defriese and Fielding, 1990). Behavioral factors, nutritional intake, environmental exposures, personality type, and the nature of social interactions all determine the qualitative and quantitative risk associated with one's health and well-being. Other issues that contribute to health risk include genetics, inheritance, prior medical treatment for disease, geography, and other elements related to sociodemography of an individual or population.

The challenge to most Americans is the unrealistic expectation for an individual to remember and to continually monitor changes in all the known risks to one's health and well-being in a proactive manner. Epidemiological studies have allowed for the identification, quantification, and classification of health risks. Using medical informatics to catalog these risks and combine them together, summarization of individual risk information will help to shape a healthy lifestyle behaviorally. In many cases, the development of clear-cut evidence of health risk precedes the development of quantification of individual risk. However, lack of specific information on the level of health risk does not prevent an individual from taking action to lower his or her risk behaviorally, even with limited scientific and evidence-based information (e.g., national cholesterol education program). Societal concern for better understanding of individual health risk is reflected in the increased attention to health promotion and disease prevention at the point of care and in other venues of healthcare delivery (Defriese and Fielding, 1990).

A tool developed in the 1970s by physicians (Robbins and Hall, 1970) to change the focus of the clinical interaction at the point of care from chronic disease to health promotion and disease prevention, called the health risk assessment (HRA), has gained popularity over the past 30 years as a means to:

- Motivate individuals to participate in health promotion and health education programs
- Enable clinicians and the healthcare delivery system to integrate a concern for disease prevention at the point of care at every clinical encounter with patients
- Enable corporate employer groups to summarize the major health problems and health risks among large groups of employees as the basis for planning corporate health promotion programs and benefit plan design
- Measure the general health patterns and behavioral risk activities of large populations to identify health risk targets for public health and educational campaigns

The health risk assessment (also called the health hazard appraisal) consists of three essential elements (Beery et al., 1986). The first element is an assessment of personal health habits (e.g., smoking, alcohol use, sleeping patterns, etc.) and risk factors based on questionnaire responses provided by the individual. This may be supplemented by biomedical measurements such as height, weight, blood pressure, cholesterol level, etc. The second element is a quantitative assessment of the individual's future risk of death and/or other adverse health outcomes from several specific causes. The final element of the health risk assessment (HRA) is a provision of educational messages and/or counseling about ways in which lifestyle changes in one or more personal risk factors might alter the risk of disease or even death.

According to Defriese and Fielding (1990), the limitations and cautions of HRA use in health promotion, health education, and clinical healthcare delivery have been identified. The most frequent and important concerns have dealt with the following issues:

- The quality of the underlying epidemiological data upon which estimates of individual health risk are based
- The limitations of available statistical methodology for estimating risk, including the problems of combining risk factors of different types into a composite personal health risk score and the methods

for adjusting for competing risks and the health consequences of lifestyle and sociodemographic characteristics of an individual

- The methodology for handling missing data in processing HRA questionnaires, since the substitution of "average values" generated by pooling population data could greatly diminish the validity and reliability of results for any given individual
- The relative risk values of general health scores that do not infer probabilities of specific health problems versus disease-specific risk estimates
- Whether the results from an HRA would be likely to be misrepresented to individuals as equivalent to a periodic health examination at the point of care by a clinician or understood to be more precise in a statistical sense than may be indicated

Improved epidemiological studies and medical informatics technology for estimating health risk, along with a substantial incremental change in relevant population- and evidence-based research, have permitted improved risk estimates for individuals completing HRAs. However, quantifiable risk estimates, when provided, often have an inherent limitation. They may include extrapolations from a limited number of studies whose populations have not included all sociodemographic groups to whom they are being applied such as minorities, elderly, and women (Defriese and Fielding, 1990).

Projected mortality risks are the hallmark outcome measurement of HRAs and this is what makes HRAs so popular in all healthcare delivery venues. However, the form of feedback an HRA provides remains a concern. These benefits should be returned in terms of absolute risk rather than in terms of qualitative statements or relative risk (Schoenback et al., 1987). The major targets of HRA use are the following: recruitment, health information, motivation, preventive health screening, clinical counseling, strategic planning, and health education program evaluation.

Utilizing these targets, HRAs today include some form of follow-up counseling session, in person or online, on an individual or group basis, along with referral to health education programs. This follow-up activity is crucial to successful outcomes management. However, the real measure of the effectiveness of HRAs in changing individual health behavior can be categorized into four major outcomes measures (Schoenback et al., 1987). The first category measures individual productivity as it relates to the workplace. It measures employee performance, absenteeism, and disability. Individual productivity can also be measured outside of the workplace and functionality and quality of life measures can be statistically categorized and reported. The second category measures overall individual and population demand for healthcare delivery services such as hospitalization rates, clinician utilization, and pharmacy utilization. The third category measures overall risk and individual risk factors such as serum glucose, serum cholesterol, weight, body mass index, smoking, alcohol consumption, cancer risk, cardiovascular risk, and total mortality risk. The fourth and final outcome measure evaluates individual health attitudes concerning beliefs about susceptibility to and severity of disease, difficulty and regularity in performing healthy activities, knowledge of disease and risk indicators, ability to modify unhealthy behavior, and efficacy of individual and clinician actions to prevent disease and promote health and well-being.

Major studies using HRAs, including large randomized trials, have been completed to establish whether HRAs are effective in stimulating healthy behavioral changes in individuals and populations (Schoenback et al., 1987). Unfortunately, these studies have not provided conclusive evidence to establish how effective HRAs are to motivating individual healthy behavioral changes. Rigorous scientific evaluation on the outcomes of a health education procedure such as the HRA is difficult because of the diversity of contexts in which the HRA is used (i.e., corporate, home, public health, etc.). In addition, behavioral interventions are highly influenced by an individual's personality traits, attitudes, level of previous knowledge on health, demand for healthcare services, and sociodemographics.

What is the ultimate outcome measure for an HRA? Many consider the HRA to be a health education tool and not a clinical intervention at the point of care between patient and clinician. With this in mind, the most appropriate outcome objective for the HRA is the transmission of health information in a personalized, relevant manner or stimulation of individual participation in health promotion programs. The HRA provides in one package a rationale, a framework for presentation of health information, an exercise that engages participants, and a personalized feedback which serves as a focused, detailed data management tool to change individual behavior for a healthy lifestyle and encourage both functionality and a high quality of life. Finally, others (Milsum, 1980) have suggested that the HRAs primary importance is in creating "a teaching moment" when a health professional as counselor and a patient as individual seeking a healthy lifestyle come together to discuss comprehensively the individual's health condition and the risks to which the individual is being exposed to on a consistent basis that may effect their quality of life and overall functionality.

DEMAND MANAGEMENT

There are several issues facing Americans who are searching for their own health and well-being. Unlimited personal healthcare needs on the part of healthcare consumers have been fueled based on sociodemographic changes consistent with an aging population, higher levels of income and education, and a general increase in knowledge for healthcare issues (Change Foundation, 2002). Technology and medical innovations allowing for genetic testing, microprocessing, and robotics have also resulted in an increase in consumer wants. Finally, easier access to healthcare information via the World Wide Web has created a personal need that has never been seen before in current healthcare delivery.

The supply side of healthcare economics is faced with controlling the rising healthcare costs through improved management of the healthcare delivery system. By controlling the supply of human resources and technology, along with the vertical and horizontal integration of healthcare services, the suppliers of health care have been struggling to keep pace with consumer's growing demand for healthcare services. Maintaining alignment between supply and demand for healthcare delivery requires improved effectiveness of care and cost efficiencies through better management and organization of healthcare services.

Utilization management, case management, evidence-based medicine, and shifting venues of healthcare delivery from high to low costing areas (e.g., inpatient services to outpatient services and home care) have assisted the demand side of economic control. Ultimately, with limited healthcare resource management capabilities and the expected increase in demand from sociodemographic and healthcare innovation trends, a strategy is needed from a population medicine approach that will have a positive effect on all facets of outcomes management including the following: clinical performance with improved health and well-being, financial performance through aligning supply and demand of healthcare services, patient satisfaction being met and channeled through healthcare consumers' expectations, enhanced quality of life and overall physical, psychological and social functionality enabled via access to technology and innovation for all.

Several definitions of demand management exist within the demand management movement. These definitions are dependent on geography and culture. From a British perspective, Pencheon (1998), defined demand management as "the process of identifying where, how, and why people demand health care and the best methods of curtailing, coping, or creating this demand such that the most cost effective, appropriate and equitable healthcare system can be developed with the public; in short, how can supply and demand for health care be reconciled fairly."

Vickery and Lynch (1995) define demand management from an American perspective:

> The support of individuals so that they may be makes rational health and medical decisions based on a consideration of benefits and risks. It is concerned with making more appropriate use of health services, not reducing it or making it cheaper-although both of these may occur.

Vickery views demand by healthcare consumers from four main perspectives:

- Morbidity—disease and illness
- Perceived need—the perception of what an individual needs to be healthy, they have the economic means to acquire it and they are willing to pay for it
- Patient preference—based on geography, culture, gender, and age
- Socioenvironmental factors—employer pressures, governmental intervention, social status, level of income, and employment.

The drivers of change in health care (e.g., aging population, technology, inappropriate use of healthcare resources, under- and uninsured individuals, chronic disease), healthcare consumer behavior, increasing choice and access for healthcare services, and alleviation of consumer fear all contribute directly to the rising interest in demand management. These factors also contribute indirectly to reducing demand for healthcare services.

Donelan (1999) reports on the measurement of public satisfaction with healthcare services in five countries: Australia, Canada, New Zealand, United Kingdom, and the United States. Over 1000 adults reported their top public concerns which included:

- Waiting times for healthcare services
- Public health and disease prevention needs
- Physician needs
- Quality of healthcare services delivered

Unfortunately, the limitations on the supply side of healthcare delivery forces demand management concepts to begin addressing these concerns.

The economic basis for developing demand management is well understood. In 2001, Levit et al. (Powell, 2003) reported that the cost of health care in the United States totaled $1.55 trillion dollars, representing almost 15 percent of the gross domestic product. The cost of health care per capita in 2002 was reported as $5,415 dollars. With current double-digit healthcare inflation, the cost per capita for healthcare services will rise to well over $8,708 dollars by 2010 (Centers for Medicare & Medicaid Services, Office of Actuary, 2002).

There is also a cultural context to understanding the basis for developing demand management programming. Rogers et al. (1998) acknowledges the need for healthcare consumer involvement for the following reasons:

- In order to promote good self care and manage demand for healthcare services better, one must understand better why, when, and for what reasons healthcare services are used by the population.
- Knowledge, culture, attitudes, experiences, and healthcare organization are the key determinants of when, why, and how people access formal healthcare services.
- The formal healthcare delivery system must build on the ways in which people already take responsibility for managing their health.
- Information that is relevant, accessible, meaningful, and integrated with other support (i.e., formal healthcare delivery) is important.
- Developing a culture in which risk, responsibility, control, and uncertainties can be quantified, discussed, and shared among all the health constituencies is a critical success factor for demand management.
- Being explicit about the limitations of the formal healthcare delivery system and the services provided improves the communication between the system and the consumer.
- Maximizing alternative ways of responding to healthcare consumers' needs is also a critical success factor for demand management.

Generally, drivers of change in healthcare delivery increase demand. However, Mark et al. (2000) identified drivers of change that can potentially decrease the demand for healthcare services: consumerism—the movement away from medical paternalism and the movement toward healthcare consumer self-reliance; information technology—the identification, storage, retrieval, and reporting of critical health information along with the proliferation of health information on the World Wide Web; and organizational behavior—culture change and alignment of incentives with all the healthcare constituencies.

Today's healthcare consumer is more knowledgeable, sophisticated, and informed than at any other time in recent history of American medicine. Because they are well-educated overall (i.e., in electronics, information technology, education) consumers no longer fear interaction with a formal healthcare delivery system, especially one-on-one with their physicians. With increasing availability of and access to personal computers, professional expertise can be harnessed and made useful for consumers in their own personal and private space. Information technology has great potential for establishing early and regular communication lines for healthcare consumers and their physicians.

Some believe (Dorwick, 1997) that patient access to explicit health information about what they can expect to receive as part of their care may create an environment at the point of care where the healthcare consumer is knowledgeable and more realistic about their expectations for outcomes after receiving healthcare services. This would result in a more manageable level of personal demand for healthcare services in the formal healthcare delivery system. Aligning demand with the capacity of an already overburdened healthcare delivery system requires changes in organizational behavior. Evidence-based medicine and population-based medicine are two current mechanisms currently changing the way healthcare services are delivered to the consumer. Both mechanisms are explicit and rationally based for clinical decision making and restore the control of healthcare services delivery into the hands of clinicians. Continuous quality improvement, outcomes management, risk analysis, and patient and medical safety programs are all receiving more attention as organizations begin to change into more consumer-oriented entities.

Forecasting future demand for healthcare services is difficult and complex at best. Population demographics and socioeconomic status, population needs and behaviors, organization and delivery of healthcare services, evolution of clinical knowledge, practice patterns and technology, geographical distribution and mix of clinicians, societal preferences, and demand for all levels of healthcare services contribute to how supply and demand for healthcare delivery will be aligned in the future. The current profile of the population will change over time with predictable trends in mortality rates, fertility rates (gender/age adjusted), migration patterns, and similar factors. The healthcare resources required will hopefully remain constant in the future.

Cost-effective methods are available and must be implemented to control how healthcare resources are used in accordance with relative levels of consumer healthcare needs. In addition to cost-effective methods of control, other economic considerations must be introduced to ensure that healthcare resources are distributed humanely and equitably and have the greatest impact on healthcare consumer needs. The ultimate goal is to channel demand by healthcare consumers into the most cost-effective, appropriate and equitable healthcare delivery system, both privately and publicly.

Healthcare consumer knowledge plays an essential role in determining the success of any demand management strategy. Demand management will be successful if it is based on a core knowledge base for healthcare consumers—their fears, understanding, and expectations; evidence-based medicine grounded in valid, reliable, relevant, and accessible research knowledge from the point of care; and current knowledge about available healthcare resources—people, facilities, and technology. It is critically important that knowledge, risk, and decisions about personal healthcare choices be shared explicitly between consumers and clinicians, among all levels of healthcare delivery, and between the community-at-large and governmental health policy makers.

The overall success for demand management strategies must begin early in life. Interventions at early stages in the life cycle have been shown to have a significant impact on both health outcomes in early life and long-term prevention of adult onset diseases (Wadsworth, 1999). From a social perspective, health-related interventions during childhood may improve resilience to stressful situations such as poverty, abuse, and malnutrition. Wadsworth (1999) describes three types of protective factors that, when demonstrated during childhood, can protect against morbidity and mortality in later life. Communication and problem-solving skills, including the ability to recruit substitute caregivers such as family relations or friends who provide affectionate ties that encourage trust, autonomy, and initiative, and relationships with others in the community-at-large who provide positive role models, reinforce and reward competencies of resilient children. Health, social behavior, socioeconomic status, and cognition are all potential benefits from such types of social support.

Demand management at the population level can be a potentially effective way of curbing future, unlimited demand for healthcare resources by the community-at-large. Health policy goals at the population level must be designed to encourage macroeconomic and cultural change (Acheson, 1995). When the health and social needs of a population are addressed proactively, then that population's health will benefit and their need, collectively and individually, for healthcare services will be minimized.

The backbone of demand management programming is medical self-care (Powell, 2001). Medical self-care refers to a decision-making process that helps healthcare consumers increase their efficiency and appropriate use of healthcare resources. In addition, medical self-care allows healthcare consumers to make better, more informed healthcare decisions such as when a real medical emergency occurs requiring immediate professional attention, when and when not to see a clinician at the point of care, when and how to provide medical self-care to oneself or another, where to appropriately access healthcare delivery services-inpatient vs. outpatient, when diagnostic testing ordered by a clinician is appropriate, and how to use shared-decision making with a clinician regarding personal diagnostic and/or treatment plan.

Teaching healthcare consumers to make better, more informed healthcare decisions will directly reduce unnecessary demand on the healthcare delivery system. It will also directly result in reduced healthcare costs, increased patient satisfaction, improved functionality, improved quality of life, and increased consumer empowerment and sense of control.

DISEASE MANAGEMENT

Under the current model of healthcare delivery in the United States, there is a steadily growing need for a systematic approach to caring for chronically diseased patients. Chronically diseased patients have their healthcare needs met with a continuum-of-care approach that involves various healthcare clinicians, treatment protocols, and points of care. This approach to disease management arose in response to the increased demand by chronically diseased patients and their families on the traditional, biomedical healthcare delivery system that would otherwise be unmanageable with the limited healthcare resources available.

Disease management programming is designed to improve both the quality and outcome of healthcare delivery. It also is interested in finding the most efficacious, effective, and efficient clinical protocols to manage chronic disease. Disease management programs are based on systematic population-based approaches to identifying patients at risk for increased morbidity and mortality, intervening with specific clinical programs that are evidence-based with well-established clinical guidelines, and measuring the clinical, financial, functional, and quality of life outcomes to provide even better clinical protocols of healthcare delivery. It is this systematizing of clinical processes leading to the prevention and early intervention of chronic, debilitating disease that separates disease management programs from traditional delivery of healthcare services by clinicians in traditional points of care.

Epstein (1996) formally defines disease management as a "systematic, population-based approach to identify persons at risk, intervene with specific programs of care, and measure clinical and other outcomes." Disease management describes a focused application of limited healthcare resources to achieve a particular health outcome in patients with chronic disease. Many disease management programs share the following characteristics: supporting the clinician–patient relationship and comprehensive plan of care, emphasizing the prevention of exacerbations and complications related to the disease, utilizing cost-efficient evidence-based medicine with clinical practice guideline implementation, and individual patient empowerment, self-care medicine, and demand management programming.

Disease management began as a direct result of the managed care movement of healthcare delivery in the United States (Neese, 2000). Coordinated primary care and preventive clinical services emerged in the early 1980s due to major concerns by payors that their members were not receiving high quality healthcare services and wide variations in clinical medical practice at the point of care existed. Wennberg (1988) documented significant variation in major surgical procedures from different regions of the country that could not be explained by sociodemographic differences or severity of the disease being treated. Others (Herzlinger, 1989) reported how managed care allowed payors to devise new financing and marketing schemes and missed opportunities to improve the quality, effectiveness, and cost-efficiency of healthcare delivery in clinical operations, human resource management, administrative oversight, and strategic health planning.

In the 1990s, high quality, cost-efficient clinical healthcare delivery was what many managed care companies strived for, allowing for natural competition to increase market share geographically. The natural tension between the quality and costs of healthcare services led all healthcare constituencies to design, develop, and implement disease management strategies.

Disease management can be viewed as an applied medical science using techniques of resource management, evidence-based medicine, clinical practice guidelines, continuous quality improvement, and medical informatics to improve the systematic, clinical processes and control of chronic disease. Using the well-known concepts of statistical process control (Wheeler and Chambers, 1992), the main goal of disease management is to decrease unexpected or special variation in the delivery of healthcare services. This ultimately improves clinical outcomes for patients and identifies the sound providers of high quality, cost-efficient clinical care.

Neese et al. (2000) describe a six-step process for disease management strategies. These strategies function as an interrelated set of tools that are applied in a specific sequence. The components of this process include:

1. Data set development
2. Establishing clinical practice guidelines
3. Determining the economic structure of disease
4. Analyzing patient segments
5. Identifying critical junctures
6. Disease management strategy implementation

The fundamental requirement for all disease management strategies is an accessible database on all individual patients. Disease management proceeds successfully as an extension of a healthcare organization's existing clinical, operations, and business data systems. Medical informatics and the development of electronic medical records require a well-coordinated process to ensure adequate identification, storage, and retrieval of necessary data points to manage care according to clinical protocols. Common patient identifiers, secure transmission, and retrieval of data are all requirements for a successful program.

Eliminating unexplained variation within the clinical process requires the design, development, and implementation of accepted algorithms of comprehensive care for the disease entity or clinical preventive service.

The algorithm provides a measurement benchmark for variation in the process. Evidence-based medicine and clinical practice guidelines have become widely available in several different formats for use throughout the public and private information channels.

Analyzing cost with respects to the delivery of systematic, population-based health care requires the use of practice management software and billing records to review the financials related to the completeness of health care delivered to patients with chronic disease. Disease-specific direct and indirect costs must be established to provide decision makers an accurate accounting of their return on investment for the programs being delivered.

Healthcare delivery is noted for providing an inordinate amount of healthcare resources to a significantly small group of the general population with chronic disease. Identifying patient segments that make substantial use of healthcare resources allows a disease management program to focus on those groups of patients that contribute the most to the costs of healthcare delivery and to improve the delivery process. In addition, focusing on the delivery of evidence-based, age-related clinical preventive services for asymptomatic individuals in the general population enables the majority of individuals access to critically important healthcare resources that promises to keep individuals healthy and fully-functional for a significant portion of their lives.

Identifying critical junctures is a step in the disease management strategy in which data show significant unexpected or special variation in either the quality or cost of the healthcare delivery process. Expected variation should be a routine occurrence as a result of sociodemographic changes, co-morbidity, and the generally accepted complexities of the healthcare delivery process. However, unexpected variation is sought out and, when discovered, dealt with aggressively.

The principles of disease management strategy implementation must be followed to ensure a successful program deployment (Neese, 2000). These fundamental principles are common sense in nature but they are often neglected in the rush for outcome results and the need for a rapid return on investment. To obtain system-wide accountability, new disease management programs should begin with common chronic diseases and clinical preventive services that have well-established and accepted evidence for what is appropriate delivery of clinical healthcare services. Small pilot programs allow for appropriate control and provide a central administrative and operational infrastructure and support for appropriate economy of scale as the scope of effort increases. As with any form of clinical programming, the clinicians must be willing to accept the effort to improve clinical processes and outcomes. In addition, clinicians must recognize the value of the program and be willing to rapidly and uniformly update clinical practice guidelines and measurement activities. Acceptance at the point of care is critical in implementing any disease management program.

Meeting the complex needs of patients with chronic disease is the single greatest challenge that organized medical practice face at the point of care. According to Wagner (1997), a multitude of surveys and audits revealed that many patients with chronic disease did not receive effective treatment, had poor disease control, and were unhappy with their care. Results of randomized control trials revealed that effective disease management programs can achieve substantially better outcomes than usual and customary health care.

The evidence suggests that a redesign of the ambulatory healthcare process at the point of care is required to improve the health care delivered to chronically diseased patients. Primary healthcare delivery at the point of care was designed to provide ready access and clinical care to patients with acute, varied problems and emphasize the following: triage and patient flow, short and effective appointments, diagnosis and treatment of symptoms and physical signs, reliance on laboratory and diagnostic investigation followed by prescription drug therapy, brief didactic patient education and training, and patient-initiated follow-up.

Patients with chronic disease and their families have special needs that are unlikely to be met by an acute healthcare delivery system and culture. As previously discussed, patients with chronic disease require planned, regular interactions with their clinical caregivers. This care must focus on functionality, quality of life, and prevention of exacerbations and complications which lead to more costly healthcare service requirements. This ongoing, comprehensive interaction includes systematic health risk assessments, attention to clinical practice and treatment guidelines, and behaviorally sophisticated support for patient self-management. These interactions require linkage through time by clinically relevant medical information systems and continuing follow-up initiated by the healthcare delivery team.

Chronic disease management programs tend to fall into two groups: targeting and case management, and comprehensive system change.

Research done by the Group Health Cooperative of Puget Sound (Wagner, 1996) led to the development of a model for improving chronic disease management. The model suggests that the patient-provider interactions that improve clinical and financial outcomes are found in formal healthcare delivery systems with a well-developed process that contains incentives for making changes at all levels. In addition, assuring behaviorally sophisticated self-management support which gives priority to increasing patients' confidence and skills and allows them to be the ultimate manager of their disease process may improve healthcare outcomes. Reorganization of healthcare team function, practices, and policies (e.g., scheduling appointments and follow up) to meet the personal needs of chronically diseased patients is a fundamental requirement for a successful program. Designing, developing, implementing, and evaluating evidence-based medicine supported at the point of care is crucial for clinicians. Through provider education, reminders, and increased interaction between primary and specialty care clinicians, enhancement of medical and clinical information systems to facilitate the design, development, implementation, and evaluation of disease registries, patient-tracking systems, and outcomes management systems will provide the final important piece of a successful chronic disease management program. This model of healthcare delivery is centered at the point of care. The locus of healthcare services being delivered remains with the personal physician who is supported by an integrated team of clinically and administratively trained staff.

Targeting and case management activities operating at the point of care follow these four major premises:

- The reduction in the cost of chronic disease is the major goal and is assumed to be associated with improvements in an individual's health and well-being.
- The best way to achieve cost-efficiencies is to focus on the highest-cost patients in the chronically diseased population.
- Primary healthcare services are not the best delivery system for chronically diseased patients.
- Patients will do better clinically and functionally if their chronic disease management is largely removed from primary healthcare delivery and delegated to a clinical case manager who coordinates their care at the point of care (Wagner, 1996).

Emphasizing quality improvement and not cost reduction maintains the access to healthcare services for chronically diseased patients. The best approach to creating cost-efficiencies is to improve overall health and well-being. In order to do this, access to healthcare delivery must be guaranteed for the chronically diseased patient. In addition, the healthcare services being provided must have a proven track record in improving clinical and functional outcomes of chronically diseased patients. Case management must do more than encourage brief hospitalizations and lower intensity follow up with mid- and lower level healthcare providers at home. Constant risk stratification of chronically diseased patients is a critical success factor for disease management programs because the health status of chronically diseased and older patients changes frequently. Chronically diseased patients benefit from periodic assessment of clinical and psychosocial status, effective clinical treatment, greater confidence and skills in self-management, and sustained follow up.

DISABILITY MANAGEMENT

Before a discussion on disability management can begin, one must review and understand what is meant by being in a state of good health and what is meant when an individual has a disease process. Health is defined by the World Health Organization (1992) as the:

> State of complete physical, emotional, and social well-being, not merely the absence of disease or infirmity . . . including intellectual, environmental, and spiritual health . . . in an active process of becoming aware of and making choices toward a more successful existence.

Health is a condition or quality of the human organism which expresses adequate functioning under given genetic and environmental conditions (e.g., individual is healthy despite challenges). Health is also thought of as efficient performance of bodily functions taking place in the face of a wide range of changing environmental conditions (e.g., expression of adaptability). Disease, on the other hand, is a pattern of responses to some form of insult or injury that results in either disturbed physiological or biochemical function or structural/morphological alteration.

A bigger issue in understanding the difference between health and disease is how the concept of "normal" is defined at the point of care. The normal state does not always indicate health as previously defined. Normal can be understood best in terms of epidemiological concepts by noting that it is an indication of the frequency of a given condition in a defined population—a reference range that has a degree of being healthy or diseased. What those in clinical medicine realize is that there are no absolutes with respects to one's state of health or disease. In fact, the disease process has four distinct stages:

1. Etiology—the cause of the disease process.
2. Pathogenesis—the mechanism behind the development of the disease process.
3. Morphologic changes—the structural changes that occur at the cellular and subcellular level.
4. Clinical significance—the physiological and biochemical changes that occur as a result of structural alterations that change the functionality of the individual.

The etiology of disease can be a direct result of a genetic alteration within the individual (congenital or acquired) and a direct result of response to one's interaction with the environment. For example, acquired causes of disease are a result of infections from microbes, fungi, viruses; nutritional deficiencies of macronutrient and micronutrient causes; chemical exposures to toxins and other like agents; physical trauma and psychosocial issues including poverty, unemployment, sanitation, immunization, living conditions, and social exclusion.

The importance of measuring disease and disease process is related to individual and population concepts of disease that include individual self-perception leading to the state of illness, professional assessment that allows for the purposeful and therapeutic interaction between patient and clinician at the point of care, and cultural norms that result in recovery from disease or ongoing illness that could lead to permanent impairment and disability. Unfortunately, disease criteria and classification of disease may change over time due real changes in occurrence, changes in names, changes in definition of "abnormal," and changes from single to multiple categories.

For clinical and evaluative purposes, disease criteria must be clearly stated and easy to measure in a standardized manner. The aim of any clinical health intervention is to cure disease completely and to alleviate pain and suffering. All clinical health evaluations must include a measurement of a disease's severity or symptoms. This is the only way to ensure that classification of an individual disease state is uniformly recorded after observation by the clinician at the point of care. Standard measures are used to compare the severity of diseases between individuals. This allows for adequate prognosis and may lead to a combination of different variables into a single scale of measurement. The dimensions of disease measurement are diagnosis, timing (i.e., acute vs. chronic), and severity (i.e., minor, incapacitating, or fatal). Understanding the severity of disease measurement could explain the chance of a patient with the disease surviving for a specified period of time, or the chance that a patient with the disease will suffer particular events related to the disease (i.e., infertility).

Typically, a simple scale for severity of symptoms is used at the point of care to determine clinical outcomes. For example, an individual patient's symptoms can be classified as mild, moderate, or severe in severity or intensity. An individual patient's clinical prognosis as a result of experiencing a disease state can also be classified for outcomes purposes as excellent, good, fair, and poor. However, traditional measures of morbidity and mortality only provide clinical information about the lowest levels of health. These traditional measures reveal little about other important aspects of an individual's or a community's level of health, including physical, psychological, and social dysfunction and disability associated with diseases, injuries, and other health problems.

Developing a composite index of overall health and well-being was needed to create data about the presence or absence of various disease and conditions (Centers for Disease Control and Prevention, 2000). In determining an individual's health status, a generic methodology can be used to predict a clinical outcome (Patrick, 1989). This generic health status is defined as a way of assessing physical, psychological, and social function that does not relate to a specific disease state. Generic health status is also a way to compare two individuals with different diseases, illnesses, or states of health and well-being. There are also disease-specific health status measurements that allow a patient's functional health to be assessed in relation to a specific disease. For example, a symptom index for patients with coronary artery disease would include the following:

1. Chest pain
   a. At rest
   b. With activity

2. Shortness of breath
   a. At rest
   b. With activity

Another way to measure health and well-being is the health status profile. The health status profile (or personal wellness profile) includes a number of dimensions and produces a range of scores representing these different dimensions. For example, exercise intensity and frequency, dietary intake, smoking, and alcohol consumption can all be quantified to predict the health status of an individual. The health status index is then developed from measuring the health status of an individual, encompassing a number of different health dimensions, and aggregating them into a single score. This score can be used to determine a health age which can then be compared to one's chronological age and match healthy behavior to a favorable health age.

From a healthcare outcomes perspective, there are a number of ways to measure the health status of an individual and provide a clinical and functional picture of that individual. This picture may be snapshots of various times of the patient's disease state or from an ongoing perspective related to one's health and well-being, and thus provides a more complete picture of an individual's impairment and disability when it is applicable to a chronically-disease patient.

The traditional measures of disease include morbidity and mortality. This includes the following sequelae after the onset of disease: cure, recovery, death, further illness, or complications. In addition to the traditional measure of disease, there are subjective, patient-based health evaluations to describe an individual's level of physical, psychological, or social functioning and their quality of life. There are a multitude of valid, reliable, and reproducible scales that can measure longitudinally a patient's subjective level of function after onset of disease or illness (e.g., SF-12, SF-36, etc.).

From a quality of life perspective, one's ability to perform activities of daily living defines one's functionality in terms of quality of life. The activities of daily living include the following categories: personal hygiene, communication, physical activity, sensory functions (five senses), hand functions, travel, sexual function, sleep hygiene, social/recreational activities, and occupational activities. An individual's ability or inability to perform these activities can be explained clinically in terms of one's level of impairment.

Impairment (AMA, 2000) is a clinically determined level of alteration of an individual's health status which results in an abnormal function of a body part or organ systems and its functioning. Impairment is the clinical loss or abnormality of psychological, physiological, biochemical, or anatomical structure of function. Conditions that interfere with an individual's activities of daily living as a result of loss of use of, or derangement of, any body part, system, or function qualify as clinical impairment. Impairment can be further defined through other measures including health-related quality of life, which is defined as the value assigned to an individual's life as modified by their physical, psychological, or social functional status.

Quality of life measurements deal with a patient's own subjective assessment of the effect of a change in health on his or her own life. It can be considered from either a generic or disease-specific health status (Patrick, 1989) and can be profiled or indexed after it is combined with the quantity of a person's remaining life to create an outcome measure and a quantifiable score (e.g., quality-adjusted life years or QALY). Quality of life is a broad and subjective term that conveys an overall sense of well-being, including aspects of happiness and satisfaction with life as a whole (Centers for Disease Control and Prevention, 2000). The primary difficulty in measuring quality of life is that the term means something different for each individual and group. A logical measurement of key concepts of quality of life have led to a more precise measurement of this conceptually complex and broad term.

Valuing the quality of life uses techniques to compare the relative values that individuals place on different states of health. It is entirely subjective and uses rating scales, magnitude estimation, and time trade-off. For example, an individual may prefer one year of perfect health to five years inability to climb stairs without dyspnea. This is a time trade-off and one that is purely subjective on the part of the individual. Additionally, it may change as an individuals' psychosocial issues change. QALY is one example of a logical measurement of key concepts of quality of life. The QALY index represents the duration of one's individual life with a particular quality of life. A numerical index that can be used to compare the outcomes of healthcare across different diseases, health states, and populations is produced.

The advantages of using an index like the QALY is that as a single index, it represents the quality, quantity, and valuation of life needed for cost-utility analyses. It can be used to compare the outcomes of different interventions applied to different diseases and different populations. Finally, it can help the process of explicit decision making, particularly with regard to prioritization of healthcare services for patients and resource allocation available in healthcare delivery.

One disadvantage of using QALY as an index of individual quality of life measure is that a ranking of states of health relies on hypothetical judgments, not objective scientific fact finding. It is the subjectivity of an individual patient's perception of health need that can lessen the validity and reliability of this measure. These judgments in turn are affected by the health and culture of those who make them. It is not always clear whose judgments should be considered, either patients, clinicians, or the community-at-large. QALY does not always provide a sufficiently sensitive measure for making clinical judgments. Different techniques for eliciting preferences give different values for the same health state. This has lead some to question the QALY and ethical objections have been raised. For example, prejudice regarding resource allocation decisions against the elderly can occur because theoretically they have less time to benefit from a decision. In addition, QALY can be used to justify failure to treat small numbers of patients with rare, expensive conditions.

An additional methodology used to measure quality of life in health days was created by the Centers for Disease Control and Prevention (CDC). It measures health-related quality of life (HRQOL) (2000). The definition of HRQOL from the CDC was "an individual's or group's perceived physical or and mental health over time." The core HRQOL Healthy Days methodology assesses a person's perceived sense of well-being through four key concept questions on: self-related health, the number of recent days (within past 30 days) when physical health was not good, the number of recent days (within past 30 days) when mental health was not good, and the number of recent activity limitation days (within past 30 days) when both physical and mental health was not good.

The number of unhealthy days provides a simple, yet comprehensive HRQOL summary measure that has been validated as a responsive index of perceived physical and mental health over time (Centers for Disease Control and Prevention, 2000). Both of these measures are critical to understanding the true health outcomes that can reflect the broad consequences of biological, psychological, social, and environmental factors affecting the lives of individuals and populations. These are truly clinical measures that can describe the level of impairment experienced by those that are studied. Moving from the clinical outcomes perspective into other aspects of outcomes management leads to a discussion on disability and disability management.

Disability can be defined as an alteration of an individual's capacity to meet personal, social, or occupational demands or statutory or regulatory requirements because of a physical or psychological impairment (American Medical Association, 2000). Disability is a relational outcome, reflecting the individual's capacity to perform a specific task or activity, contingent on the environmental conditions in which they are to be performed (Brandt, 1997). Disability is context specific. It is not inherent in the individual who possesses impairment, but a function of the interaction of the individual and his/her environment. An individual can have a disability in performing a specific task at work but not have a disability in any other social role (i.e., parent, sibling, friend, neighbor, etc.).

Disability management requires a complete understanding of an individual's impairment from a clinical perspective in combination with information about an individual's skill's, education, job history, family history, adaptability, age, and environmental stressors as it relates to performing a specific work or social task. The assessment of these factors in total can provide a more realistic picture of the effects of an individual's impairment on the ability to perform complex work and social activities. If adaptations can be made to the environment, the individual may not be disabled from performing the specific activity or activities in question.

For example, an individual with a healthy back experiences a work-related injury after lifting a 100-pound box from floor to waist. The individual becomes a patient and is seen by his family doctor for evaluation of his low back injury. After a complete history and physical examination, the clinician identifies that the patient cannot extend his back without severe pain, the patient has several neurological deficits in his left lower leg (i.e., loss of a simple reflex at the knee), and is unable to work without a limp. The clinician orders a diagnostic study (e.g., magnetic resonance imaging) of the patient's lumbar spine. A herniated disc in the lower lumbar region is diagnosed; this explains the decreased range of motion in the patient's back and his inability to use his left leg (i.e., impairment). After an appropriate amount of time and treatment for this condition, the patient is clinically assessed as to whether he can return to the jobsite and lift the same 100-pound box that caused his injury. The patient's clinician will not allow the patient to return to the workplace and lift 100-pound boxes without some form of mechanical assistance (i.e., mechanical lift). The patient's workplace does not have anything to help him mechanically lift this box and henceforth, he cannot return to his job. Thus, the patient now has a disability. When and if the workplace makes a mechanical lift available to the patient, the patient can return to the workplace to lift 100-pound boxes from floor to waist. At this point, from a disability management perspective, the patient no longer has a disability with respects to this specific activity.

Disability management is primarily a work-related phenomenon and has become a major focus for human resources departments in many corporate settings today. Compliance with the Americans with Disabilities Act (ADA, 1990), civil rights legislation signed into law in 1990 by President George H.W. Bush, has resulted in many questions for employers pertaining to individual work disability and capacity in the workplace. A brief discussion presented in the AMA *Guides to Evaluation of Permanent Impairment* (2000), follows. This illustrates the dynamics behind disability management in today's workplace as it applies to population-based medicine and outcomes management.

The ADA was intended to provide a clear, concise and comprehensive national mandate to end discrimination against all individuals with disabilities. It was also intended to allow entry into mainstream America both economically and socially for people with disabilities. The ADA protects disabled Americans in all venues such as employment, government service rights, and access to public accommodations (e.g., healthcare services, lodging, transportation, etc.).

The ADA defines disability using the following three basic criteria: a physical or mental impairment that substantially limits one or more of major life activities of an individual, a record of impairment, or a record of being regarded as having impairment. A person needs to meet only one of the three criteria in the above definition to gain the protection of the ADA against discrimination. Clinical input is required for the first two criteria and the third criterion is more of an administrative determination. To be deemed disabled for purposes of protection by the ADA, an individual must have a physical or mental impairment that substantially limits one or more major life activities. A physical or mental impairment could be any biochemical, physiological or psychological disorder or condition, cosmetic disfigurement, or anatomical loss that affects one or more of the following organ systems:

1. Neurologic
2. Special sense organs
3. Musculoskeletal
4. Respiratory including speech organs
5. Reproductive
6. Cardiovascular
7. Hematologic
8. Lymphatic
9. Digestive
10. Genitourinary
11. Dermatologic

ENDOCRINE

Conditions that are temporary, such as pregnancy, and conditions that are not considered to be severe are not impairments under the ADA. For example, old age, sexual orientation, smoking, and current illegal drug use do not qualify for protection under this act. On June 23, 1999, (Sutton v. United Airlines, 1999), the Supreme Court clarified the definition of disabled stating that individuals who function normally with aids such as glasses or medication could not generally be considered disabled despite their physical impairment.

Major life activities, as referred to in the act, include basic activities that the average person in the community-at-large can perform with little or no difficulty including caring for oneself, manual tasks, hearing, walking learning, speaking, breathing, working, and reproduction. These major life activities do not have to occur frequently or be a part of daily life. An individual must be presently or perceived to be (not potentially or hypothetically), substantially limited to demonstrate a disability. It is difficult to determine if impairment substantially limits a major life activity. The nature, extent, duration, impact, and effect of an individual's state of impairment are all considerations in assessing the substantiality of the limitations. Determining how much a limitation of a major life's activity results in a disability depends on the interaction between the remaining functional abilities of the individual and the possible types of accommodation being sought.

The key to determining how an individual may require ADA protection is performing a comprehensive clinical evaluation at the point of care by a clinician, usually a physician. The physician is responsible for informing an employer or other requesting agent about an individual's abilities and limitations. It is then the employer's or the appropriate agent's responsibility to accept the clinical information determined at the point of care about impairment and identify and determine if reasonable accommodations are possible to enable an individual's performance of essential job and other social activities. The functional outcome analysis at the point of care is critical for determining protection under the ADA.

From a population medicine approach, disability management has been relegated to the domain of large and medium size employers managing their employee productivity and absenteeism. In the early 1980s, large employer groups needed to protect themselves against rapidly rising healthcare costs, worker compensation, and other disability-related expenses that had risen dramatically in the 1970s (Galvin, 1986). Because of their size and the need to reduce rising healthcare costs, large employers in the United States developed initiatives to better manage their ill and injured employees in hopes of maintaining the health and productivity of valuable human resources.

Beginning in the 1990s, proponents of disability management in the workplace stressed the need to fully coordinate all disability-related programs (i.e., worker compensation, short term disability, long term disability, and medical care) to realize the healthcare cost savings required to maintain profitability in their marketplace (Schwartz, 1984). In the absence of an integrated approach to health and disability, employers experienced cost shifting among their internal disability management programs without a real reduction in overall healthcare costs. For example, Butler, Gardner, and Gardner (1998) reported that when claimants moved from traditional medical care or absenteeism to worker compensation, the "moral hazard" of unaccountable cost shifting resulted in increased benefits use by the injured/ill employee and reduced the overall productivity for the employer.

Despite an attempt to fully integrate disability management programs, little has been achieved in resolving disability claims of long duration. The private employer sector in the United States assists individuals in obtaining Social Security Disability Income (SSDI) benefits (Schwartz, 1984). Thus, when private employers fail to accommodate injured/ill employers and return them to meaningful work, the final solution is one of cost-shifting to public disability programs.

There has been an incremental change in the migration of private sector disabled employees to the Social Security rolls. Early intervention with aggressive worksite rehabilitation became the mainstay for employer-sponsored disability management. The ultimate outcome was to prevent individuals passing from productive work/life activity to public disability programs (Jarviskowski and Lahelma, 1980). Unfortunately, some portion of disabled employees continue to migrate to public sector disability systems (Burkhauser, Butler, and Kim, 1995). The United States General Accounting Office (U.S. GAO) has documented a significant increase in the number of public disability beneficiaries every year since 1982. Factors contributing to this problem include the emergence of new types of disability participants, structural changes in the labor market, the decline of availability of employer-based insurance benefits, extensions of the length of time over which benefits are continued, and the lack of an effective return-to-work focus (Ross, 1996).

According to Ross (1996), during the 1990s, only 1 in 500 SSDI beneficiaries left the disability rolls to return to their workplace. The U.S. GAO estimated that nearly three billion dollars could be saved in lifetime cash benefits for every one percent of working-age beneficiaries who return to work. Private sector employers with successful integrated disability management programs emphasizing return to work could help beneficiaries return to work.

The costs of disability and the growing rate of participation in disability benefit programs (especially among younger, working age applicants) are threatening factors to both public and private sector budgets (Reno, Mashow, and Gradison, 1997). These trends have brought a renewed attention to the need to reduce unnecessary work disability, to provide more effective and more timely interventions for injured/ill workers, and to design benefits policies that create stronger incentives to control costs and achieve positive outcomes whenever possible (Reno, 1997; Rupp and Stapleton, 1998).

According to McMahon et al. (2000), there exists a natural tendency by an insurer at each level of economic benefit to transfer responsibility for payment to disabled workers to another source. When this is possible, it represents the most financially expedient solution to the problem of ongoing exposure and cost to the insurer and the employers they represent. This represents a trend symptomatic of a non-integrated disability management approach in which potential cost savings and productivity gains associated with proactive integrated disability management programs are lost. A cottage industry of claimant representation firms has developed to expedite the movement of disabled workers through various levels of disability benefits and ultimately to the public disability payment system (i.e., SSDI). In terms of financial outcomes, this represents a cost shifting arrangement as opposed to a cost-aversion strategy for benefit planning. Employers and insurers should aim to screen all long-term disability claimants carefully to ensure that all reasonable efforts at return to work are exhausted.

To improve the healthcare outcomes of disability management, the progression of disability benefits (PODB) phenomenon must be halted or revised. The PODB phenomenon can be defined as the progression of workers with work-limiting disabilities moving through a system of economic disability benefits which ultimately results in their placement into the Social Security disability system. To reverse this phenomenon, employers can no longer abdicate the management of workplace disability issues to an insurer or third party administrator.

Shrey and Lacerte (1997) refer to this abdication of employer responsibility as the "lack of employer empowerment." In addition, a fully integrated (i.e., worker compensation, short term disability, long term disability, medical care) disability management program with aggressive return-to-work support must be instituted in all size employers, not just the medium to large size organizations. Because employees change jobs and companies based on the economic stability of the marketplace, all employer groups need to avail themselves of this progressive disability management concept to mitigate direct and indirect loss of human resources and therefore lost revenue and productivity. Other tools available to the employers include benefit plan design and aggressive, meaningful return-to-work programming for disabled workers regardless of the etiology of their injury or illness (i.e., occupational and non-occupational). This can be accomplished in all venues of employment, private and public, including those workplaces that operate with collective bargaining.

Measuring the outcomes of an employer's disability management program is key to identifying core success factors for future design, development, and implementation of better disability management programming. Historically, traditional indicators of effective disability management have included employee return-to-work rates, incidence and duration of absence from the workplace, worker productivity, employee satisfaction, and benefit cost reduction.

Although these outcome measurements demonstrate the value of a disability management program, McMahon et al. (2000) note these traditional indicators of outcomes are independent measures, lack powerful information, and have been rarely studied in a longitudinal manner. McMahon et al. (2000) also note that the effectiveness of disability management programs could be measured by utilizing the following PODB indicators:

- The early identification of persons at high risk to advance through PODB.
- The ability of disability management programs to interrupt the PODB phenomenon.
- The impact of disability management programs on each level and type of disability benefit including worker compensation, short term disability, long term disability, and medical care.
- The employer's experience with disability in longitudinal, economic (i.e., direct and indirect costs) terms.
- The potential to prevent premature dependence of disability claimants on public disability income.
- Measuring the productivity gains associated with retention and/or re-employment of disabled workers.

As previously mentioned, disability management is an approach generated by employers to control rising costs of disability incurred during the 1980s and 1990s. The best and most complete definition of disability management is the following (Akabas, Gates, and Galvin, 1992):

> . . . a workplace prevention and remediation strategy that seeks to prevent disability from occurring or, lacking that, to intervene early following the onset of disability using coordinated, cost-conscious, quality rehabilitation service that reflects an organizational commitment to continued employment of those experiencing functional work limitations. The remediation goal of disability management is successful job maintenance, or optimum timing for return to work.

The concept of integrated disability management (IDM) evolved out of the above definition. Linking the entire administration of healthcare delivery services, benefits, and case management components so they complement one another is the key to improving disability outcomes. By using a comprehensive IDM program, employers can avoid the conflicting philosophies, redundant administrative costs, and constant turf battles between departments in human resources administering different benefits. According to

Flynn (2000), IDM programming in its basic form coordinates occupational and nonoccupational disability benefits, absence management, and paid leave programs with the focus on rapid, early return to work that is productive and meaningful to both the employer and employee.

Some IDM programs can also provide comprehensive, corporate health management by coordinating healthcare services to their employees including traditional healthcare delivery including physician care and hospitalization, employee assistance programs for substance abuse, workplace conflict and absence management, behavioral health programs, chronic disease management, disease prevention and health promotion, and medical case management services.

The overall success of IDM programming and comprehensive, coordinated corporate health management looks to improve the overall health and well-being of the workforce, to establish a rapid and efficient return to work program for disabled employees, to decrease the administrative burdens on the employer, and to provide a seamless set of health benefits for workers with disabling injuries and illnesses.

The Washington Business Group on Health (WBGH), in conjunction with the consulting firm Watson Wyatt, surveyed employers in 2000 and discovered that employers were adopting IDM programs to stem the rising costs of health care, reduce absenteeism, increase worker productivity, manage the increasing prevalence of chronic disease among an aging workforce, and attract and retain employees. This same survey identified best practices of IDM programming that improved the outcomes in companies who used them as part of their disability management activities regularly. For example, absence rates for employees were three times higher among firms that did not use IDM best practices (Watson Wyatt, and WBGH, 2000).

There are five best IDM practices that have been identified to correlate highly with reduced healthcare costs to employers.

1. The first practice is designing, developing, and implementing a modified-duty, return-to-work program. This program is an established, measurable activity that facilitates the rapid, efficient return to work of injured and ill employees in a modified, productive form for any employee with a disability regardless of the etiology or applicable benefits system.

2. The second is the utilization of disability case management. In an IDM program, a case manager with clinical and/or rehabilitative

skills navigates the disabled employee through the medical and administrative bureaucracy with the ultimate goal of rapid, efficient, and safe return to work in a productive capacity.

3. The third identifies one point of administrative contact who files all occupational and nonoccupational benefit claims.

4. The fourth practice is to assign a single manager or department responsible for all occupational and nonoccupational benefits plans.

5. The fifth and final practice is in increasing the involvement of the disabled employee's supervisor in the workplace to assist and facilitate the rapid, efficient, and safe return to productive work in hopes of reducing recidivism and longer periods of time away from work.

From a healthcare outcomes management and planning perspective, Danczyk-Hawley et al. (2000) discuss the need to evaluate disability management programs from three major areas:

- Program effectiveness—does the DM practice lead to a reduction in the number of disability claims and increase the number of disabled employees who return to work rapidly, efficiently and safely?

- Benefit plan design adequacy—are the right incentives provided within the benefit plan design to encourage disabled employees to return to work quickly versus dependency on disability benefits for extended periods of time?

- Claims administrative capabilities—are disability claims where a disabled employee could be returned to work recognized early enough or are claimants needlessly progressing into higher disability benefit levels?

It is quite evident that disability management programs can improve return-to-work outcomes and reduce the PODB and dependence on SSDI. This ultimately results in greater workplace flexibility and reduced benefits costs to the employer. Incorporating disability management programs into the workplace will pave the way for improved employment prospects for people with disabilities (Danczyk-Hawley, 2000). In a survey of its members, the Washington Business Group on Health reported that the presence of disability management programs can contribute to increased workplace accommodations and enhanced acceptance of employees with disabilities (Bruyere, 2000). Employers with IDM programs indicated that as a result of instituting an IDM program, the following improvements were noted resulting in greater acceptance of disabled employees in the workplace:

- Successful implementation and compliance with the Americans with Disabilities Act
- Greater supervisor awareness of the workplace accommodation process
- Establishment of an organizational structure for workplace accommodations for disabled employees
- Recognition of the importance of medical information confidentiality in compliance with HIPAA

CONCLUSION

Population-based medicine requires a multidisciplinary approach to designing, developing, implementing and evaluating healthcare service delivery to specific populations in need of healthcare goods and services. Focusing on the health of the population, improvements in the quality of life and functionality are key outcome measures. Identifying successful interventions at the population level allows for this information to be applied at the individual level. Understanding health enhancement; risk management; disease demand and disability management enables all constituents of the population-at-large to benefit and increase the likelihood of having positive healthcare outcomes, regardless of whether they are the professionals delivering the care or patients receiving the care.

CHAPTER 13

Environmental Health Management

ECOSYSTEMS AND POPULATION HEALTH

The growing human population, energy-intensive technology, and consumption of natural resources are overloading the earth's ability and capacity to absorb, replenish, and repair its ecosystems. These environmental issues endanger the overall health and well-being of humans everywhere on the planet because of an increasingly damaged life-support system. Population health and its tenets (as discussed in Chapter 12) are in grave danger and cannot be sustained if the world's natural ecological systems degrade, decay, and become dysfunctional. A.J. McMichael (1993) provides an insightful look into how changing ecosystems affect the health and well-being of populations. These changes will lead to a significant impact on population-based medicine and outcomes management and planning. The following is a synopsis of his discourse on the ecosystems and population health management.

The most serious potential consequences of global environmental change are the degradation, decay, and dysfunction of the earth's life-support systems. As life evolved over time, the earth's environmental characteristics have changed considerably. The earth's lower atmosphere's composition changed, the stratospheric ozone's composition was formed from oxygen produced by plants, the soil's composition was created by oxidation, and plants, forests, and microbes sped the recirculation of rainwater. Life's genetic diversity conferred a capacity for adaptive change. However, McMichael points out that life-supporting mechanisms are starting to degrade, decay, and become dysfunctional as the cumulative global impact of human activity escalates.

It is a fundamental fact that the earth's natural life systems provide the essential life-support services that enable living organisms to remain healthy with the ability to proliferate future generations. Today's global environmental changes such as climate change, ozone layer depletion, land degradation, and loss of biodiversity will have profound effects on the health and well-being of human populations now and in the future. In fact, as the focus today has shifted away from sustained, natural development for all ecosystems to individual, personal economic development, the future generation's prospects earning potential has been severely compromised due to the decay, degradation, and dysfunction of the earth's life-support mechanisms.

It is intuitively evident that human beings cannot live apart from nature. The emerging risk to human populations' health and well-being do not arise from local environmental hazards. Rather, according to McMichael (1993), the risks arise from the decay, degradation, and dysfunction of natural ecosystems. These risks are created because human beings are exceeding the biosphere's carry capacity. In other words, humans are overloading the earth's metabolic capacity to absorb, replenish, and restore its life-support mechanisms.

It is the impairment of productivity and stability of the earth's life-support systems that is of critical and extreme importance to improving the health outcomes of all populations. To illustrate this point, McMichael describes environmental issues related to the combustion of fossil fuels. Initial concerns related to fossil fuel combustion were over the resultant local pollution by toxic gaseous emissions which at smog concentrations resulted in human illness and death. Subsequent to this crisis, our energy-intensive society became concerned over the possibility of a fossil fuel shortage, especially a crude oil production shortage. Now, even with emission control standards and proven reserves of fossil fuels for generations to come, the problems faced by humans are related to loading the atmosphere with a heat-trapping gas, carbon dioxide, that eventually will disrupt many of the biosphere's natural cycles, processes, and conditions on which humans depend for life-support.

Over the last 10,000 years of human development on earth, two major categories of environmental issues have been overcome. The first of these issues has been the problem of controlling and surviving contagious infectious diseases. The second of these issues is a result of exposure to toxic chemicals produced from increasing industrial activity. By limiting, controlling, and conquering exposures to contagious infectious diseases and toxic chemicals (along with toxic physical and biological agents), humans have adapted and flourished for several generations.

More recently, the issues that confront human populations environmentally are quite different. The convergence of population ecosystems, population pressures, land degradation, climate change, groundwater depletion, and genetic impoverishment of breeding stock to cause significant food and water shortages in the twenty-first century has become a major concern politically, economically, and socially throughout the planet. The possible impacts on today's and tomorrow's human population related to direct and indirect environmental effects, immediate and delayed environmental effects, and local and global environmental effects will be devastating to healthcare outcomes management and planning.

The current trends in global population growth, the disappearance of a middle class of citizens in developed countries, and the associated global disruptions to the atmosphere, soil, and groundwater are well documented. Yet, little is known about the intimate relationship between ecological systems and the health and well-being of human populations. The daily maintenance of individual health and well-being is determined by immediate circumstances, family history, behavioral and lifestyle activities, employment, locally-circulating contagious infectious agents, and overall luck. In developed societies, it is a well established process to focus on individual health and disease eradication without developing a similar perspective for the population as a whole. The ecological issues of population health are well below the radar screen politically, socially, and economically.

Today, the potential adverse health outcomes of global environmental decay, degradation, and dysfunction are usually distant in both time and place. It is human nature, according to McMichael, to deal with current health crises rather than to project out into the future. Unfortunately, having a short-term gain psychosocially is the very process that jeopardizes the long-term needs of human beings and their ecosystems. McMichael points out that what is needed is a capacity to override local ecological constraints and develop a biopsychosocial approach that reestablishes an ecologically sustainable way of life for future generations. How to accomplish this goal is the debate that is taking center stage today locally, regionally, nationally, and globally.

To reestablish an ecologically sustainable way of life a well-understood model that is simple to design, develop, and implement is necessary. To understand the ecological framework required to meet this objective, the relationship between ecosystems and population health must be defined. First, the environment is that part of the earth that surrounds the population. Modern societies in developed countries refer to the environment as a platform for human activity, not really a place where people live. Over time, humans have slowly but surely distanced themselves from nature. As a result, mankind stands outside the framework of nature, and has little regard for the underlying ecological dimensions of our existence; our actions and behaviors are dictated by and valued by current culture. However, the essence of the ecological framework, or ecosystem, is an obligatory interdependence between living organisms and their biopsychosocial environment.

An ecosystem is a closed system of dynamic, interdependent relationships between living organisms and their biological, physical, and chemical environment. Other than isolated small islands, most ecosystems become continuous with adjacent and adjoining ecosystems. In total, all of the earth's ecosystems occupy what is called the "biosphere." The biosphere refers to the domain on and near the earth's surface where the current conditions enable solar energy to produce the geochemical, geophysical, and geobiological changes necessary to sustain and support life. The biosphere comprises all living organisms along with the lower atmosphere, the hydrosphere, and the upper lithosphere.

Ecosystems provide the framework that allows solar energy to be captured and funneled through a hierarchy of life-forms on earth. Planet life provides the means to capture solar energy and convert it to chemical energy. Animals feed on the plants and other animals. The quest for food is the central organizing principle of life within every ecosystem. All ecosystems have mechanisms by which nutrients are retained and recycled and by which water and respirable gases are disseminated and replenished. Life does not create new matter. Instead, it recycles nutrients, using solar energy to build and maintain the temporary biological structures. Each of the atoms and sub-atomic particles in our body is on short-term lease from nature's warehouse.

Through the coevolution of species, ecosystems acquire self-stabilizing life-support mechanisms and a dynamic, yet delicate internal balance. Within a stable ecosystem, species learn to cohabitate and share the nutrients required to sustain these life-supporting mechanisms. However, each ecosystem has a carrying capacity unique to itself. That is, all things being equal, all living organisms flourish interdependently and sustain their existence as long as there is plentiful nutrition that can be acquired, stored, used, and recycled to maintain the balance of life-support in the ecosystem. Unfortunately, evolution occurs in response to current ecological opportunity, not in relation to future needs of the ecosystem. It is this here and now characteristic that threatens ecosystem sustainability. Those ecosystems with well-buffered stability and balance will survive the longest with the most efficiency for life-support.

An ecosystem cannot yield substantial and sustained increases in materials and energy to the human species without depriving other species and eventually causing damage to the productivity and variability of the ecosystem. The problem is not just overdrawing against nature's capital assets, but of harming the productivity and viability of nature's life-support mechanisms. Within the established ecological framework, overloading or exceeding the capacity of an ecosystem will ultimately degrade, decay, and dismantle the ecosystem's life-support systems.

Current economic doctrine and a free-market mentality dismiss the costs incurred by natural and human resource depletion, pollution, ecological disruption, and health impairment as a means to increase economic growth and productivity. This ultimately leads to and results in the increase of personal, individual monetary wealth and prosperity. Therefore, expending valuable environmental capital assets in the name of economic growth and productivity has become an acceptable way of life in many developed and developing countries today. Historically, humans have been able to acquire more environmental capital including fertile soils, freshwater, forests, and fossil fuels by moving into new ecosystems and repeating the process as required to replenish their natural resources. Unfortunately, *exponential* growth of the population while experiencing *arithmetic* growth of nutrients has begun to change the focus of economics from rationally allocating competitively sought after natural resources to searching for mechanisms to sustain valuable, ecological life-support in the face of finite, exhaustible natural resources. This will undoubtedly create risk to the long-term health and well-being of human populations as the capacity of natural life-support systems is eroded.

It is clear that environmental hazards are changing with the disruption of the stability and productivity of the biosphere's life support mechanisms. This change poses a qualitatively different type of health hazard to human populations. Global environmental changes, as previously discussed, may cause serious or irreversible changes in ecosystems so that current and future populations will be unable to survive and flourish. Variations in personal, individual health behavior and local cultures within the population may contribute to this phenomenon, but it is the actual stability of the ecosystems that will ultimately determine the healthcare outcomes of populations. Humans are an integral and balancing factor in the health and well-being of all ecosystems.

Historically, the major influences upon the health of populations has been those that derive from cultural values and practices, material standard of living, social organization, and characteristics of the physicochemical environment. These influences set the parameters within which the health of populations exists. Therefore, population health reflects population circumstances. It is also within these parameters that the health of individuals is largely determined by personal behaviors and circumstances. Ambient environmental exposures such as the quality of air, water, and food, along with the presence of contagious infectious diseases, have also been fundamental determinants of population health. Humans can adapt to varied environments, control aspects of the environment, and increase their productivity within and among ecosystems. However, human populations cannot live without a well-balanced ecological framework that maintains clean air, safe water, adequate food, tolerable temperatures, stable climate, biodiversity, and protection from solar ultraviolet radiation.

Human's health and well-being has long been affected by the ambient environment including the airs and waters. As urban development has progressed, the health status of populations has also been affected. This is the basis for using the biopsychosocial approach in healthcare delivery systems. Within the past few decades, an ecological framework has emerged which relates long-term population health outcomes management and planning to the carrying capacity of earth's life-support systems. An appreciation for human culture has recently grown; human cultures have introduced many types of evolutionary changes that have distorted ecological relationships and reduced the carrying capacity of ecosystems to support the health and well-being of the human population. The power of human adaptation and ingenuity has allowed populations to modify, defer, and even ignore the seriousness of this unending dilemma. However, as McMichael points out, "it is in the nature of ecological systems that debts are finally called in."

History has provided many examples of human civilizations that have declined as their ecological life-support mechanisms have eroded. Contagious infectious disease epidemics that come and go have reflected changes in human ecosystems over the centuries. Population health has been influenced by changes in security—the amount and type of food available for consumption by humans. As humans have tried to increase their food sources for better survival, diseases of affluence and excess have appeared in longer-living adult populations of developed countries.

The earth's biosphere is a closed and finite system. By the end of the twenty-first century, the human population will grow from around five and a half billion today to between 10 and 14 billion by 2100. As the human population grows, the threat of natural and human resource wars will escalate. Desperate search for drinking water, arable land, energy, and nutrition will undoubtedly affect populations globally. The control of human population growth is paramount so the carrying capacity of the earth's biosphere is not exceeded. Politics, social issues, and economics between and within countries must focus on creating a more equitable sharing of the earth's natural and human resources.

In the discussions about the earth's biosphere and its viability for the future, a concern about the conservation of non-renewable natural resources is often raised. One non-renewable resource is the biodiversity of all currently living species and the complex ecosystems in which they habitat. Species, and particularly their gene pool, are not retrievable once they are lost. This biodiversity of the species is a fundamental resource in many ways. Basically, humans consume the phenotype (i.e., the mature individual with its chemical constituents), while the genetic information from the genotype is applied. The many species consumed by humans are a source of food, socially useful chemicals, and materials used for human survival. Genetic variation is the source of nature's basic adaptive capacity. For the same reason, humans exploit it as the source of genetic stock, both as new species and as genetic variants of current species for improving the food supply. Support for the maintenance of biodiversity can only lead to a better, richer existence for all living organisms.

Ultimately this improves the health and well-being of human populations and creates a stronger ecological framework supporting the life-support mechanisms needed today and for future generations to come.

ENVIRONMENTAL HEALTH MANAGEMENT

As previously discussed, environmental health management encompasses all aspects of daily life. From an outcomes management and planning perspective, environmental improvements have both a direct and indirect impact on healthcare delivery related to quality, cost, access, and service. The quality of the environment and the nature of economic development must be balanced to achieve individual and population health and well-being. Achieving this balance requires all economic development to meet the healthcare delivery service needs of its sustaining population. In addition, a solid framework of ecological sustainability is paramount to ensure that nature's life support mechanisms may be maintained without being damaged or destroyed.

Health and well-being has been defined in previous chapters within the context of the biopsychosocial approach to healthcare delivery. Achieving a healthy lifestyle requires an active process of becoming aware of and making healthier behavioral choices for a more successful existence. The availability of natural and human resources to meet basic human needs is paramount to this active process. In addition, protection from biological, physical, and chemical hazards is required to achieve an individual sense of security and well-being.

The World Health Organization (1993) has also developed a comprehensive definition for environmental health. According to the WHO definition, environmental health comprises those aspects of human health including quality of life and functionality that are determined by physical, biological, chemical, social, and psychological factors in the environment. This definition also refers to the theories and concepts of assessing, correcting, controlling, and preventing potentially adverse factors to the health and well-being of present and future generations.

There is an interdependent relationship between human activities, the physical environment, and the biological environment that results in a healthy population (WHO, 1992). Human activities are comprised of those activities that require both active and passive behavioral actions.

These human activities may include the following: agricultural activities, industrial activities, energy production, waste management, water management, urbanization, human services, and health and environmental protection. The physical environment comprises the soil and its chemical composition, air, water, and climate. The biological environment includes the type and distribution of the following: ecosystems, habitats, flora, fauna, pathogens, reservoirs, and vectors. In order to balance the interdependent relationships among human activities, the physical and biological environments, the principle of respect for nature and the control of environmental degradation should guide the pursuit for individual and population health and well-being (Landon, 2000).

Sustainable development is a concept that enables the pursuit of long-term health and well-being (Landon, 2000; WHO, 1997). This concept is when the needs of the individual and population of the present generation are met without compromising the ability of future generations to meet their same needs. Specifically, sustainable development is the provision of basic necessities, food, employment, shelter, and health care for all of the population in a manner that prejudices none and preserves their ecosystems, the biosphere, and all of their natural resources. The basic requirements for achieving health and well-being include clean air, safe and sufficient water, adequate and safe food supplies, safe and peaceful settlements, and a stable global environment.

Why do health professionals, both administrative and clinical, need to have a basic knowledge of environmental health? It is with this knowledge that health professionals are empowered to identify and correct environmental health hazards and risks to individuals and the community-at-large, analyze the technical and biopsychosocial solutions for the reduction of human exposure to biological, physical, and chemical toxins, and lessen the potential health impacts that lead to adverse healthcare outcomes clinically, functionally, financially, and humanitarily.

SYSTEMS MODEL FOR ENVIRONMENTAL CHANGE

For the health and well-being of populations to flourish now and in the future, principles and practices of environmental change need to be designed, developed, and implemented. A model has been proposed by

Kuby et al. (1998) that establishes a linear, systematic approach to environmental changes to embrace the biopsychosocial approach to healthcare delivery. This model of change identifies a number of human driving forces that initiates the beginning of environmental change. The human driving forces are the underlying political, social, and economic conditions which influence the effects of the environment on healthcare outcomes. For example, when the price per barrel of oil is low, production of oil processing increases and more petroleum products are available to the public for consumption. This leads to environmental increases in the by-products of combustion which ultimately leads to changes in the ozone layer and respiratory difficulties for those with chronic lung disease.

After the human driving forces are initiated, human activities begin to change. For instance, the supply and demand for goods and services in all sectors of the economy, especially in industry and household consumption begins to change. Human activities that are changing will result in behaviors that can initiate environmental changes. For example, the general use of energy, goods and services distribution, and biological manipulation are contributors to the development of global environmental change. Finally, there are human and natural consequences that follow environmental changes which most recently have had an adverse impact on populations as a whole including ozone layer depletion, the loss of ecosystems, climate change, the loss of biodiversity, and land degradation.

As the systems model of environmental change progresses, other driving forces may be identified to lead to positive changes in healthcare outcomes for the community-at-large. These additional driving forces include urbanization, technology development, sociopolitical reforms, economic development, and cultural value change. For example, urbanization creates distinctive population dynamics as a driving force for environmental change because the sociodemographic changes that occur during urbanization forces the public and private sector to address issues related to healthcare outcomes management (i.e., healthcare resource distribution, natural resource consumption, waste management, and other environmental health management issues). Another example is how technology and scientific development creates new hazards and risks that need to be identified and overcome. These new hazards and subsequent risks can change patterns of human consumption and production through large scale use of natural and human resources.

The importance of these driving forces within the Systems Model of Environmental Change is that the driving forces identified may provide opportunities to mitigate or increase environmental health threats. Of course, the combination of public and private interventions can also have a significant impact, either positively or negatively, via legislation, regulation, and administration. How can this model be used to identify environmental health threats and mitigate these threats from a healthcare outcomes perspective? The following example illustrates the answer.

A factory is polluting the community within which it is located with dioxin, a known carcinogenic chemical that has been established scientifically and clinically to pose a health risk to the community-at-large. To identify and mitigate the driving forces behind the environmental threat to the local community, several questions are formed using the Systems Model of Environmental Change:

1. How is the population of the local community structured?
2. What is the socioeconomic status of the local community?
3. What technology and scientific development is required to deal with the carcinogenic pollutant?
4. What is required to deal with the political, social, and economic considerations posed by this exposure to the local community?

By answering these few questions, a linear systematic approach identifies the human driving forces, human activities, environmental changes, and the human and natural consequences posed by this environmental threat. The issues are more effectively resolved to mitigate harm to the local community now and for the future generations to come.

HAZARD VS. RISK

Identifying environmental threats to the health and well-being of populations within the context of healthcare outcomes management and planning requires valid, reliable, and responsive measures of risk. As previously discussed, health risk assessments quantify risk factors (i.e., cholesterol level, alcohol use, smoking, blood glucose) that lead to individual chronic disease states with reduced functionality as the disease state progresses.

Measuring environmental threats may be done both qualitatively and quantitatively (Landon, 2000; WHO, 1997). Hazards in the environment are qualitative measures of factors or exposures that adversely affect the health and well-being of populations. Hazards identify the potential of an environmental agent to harm individuals or populations if the exposure is above a critical level of toxicity. Environmental risks are used to quantitatively measure the probability that an adverse event will occur. Risk in general is the probability that an individual will develop disease or even die within a stated period of time or age after an exposure has been established to an environmental threat. Risk is a quantitative measure of probability that a healthcare outcome will occur after an individual or a population has been exposed to a specified, critical amount of hazard.

Hazards can be classified as either traditional or modern. Traditional hazards include:

- Lack of access to safe water
- Inadequate or poor quality housing
- Inadequate basic sanitation
- Food contamination with pathogens
- Dietary deficiencies
- Contagious infectious disease vectors
- Inadequate solid waste disposal
- Natural disasters

Traditional hazards are often realized in societies where development is slow or non-existent.

Modern hazards include:

- Water pollution related to intensive industry or agriculture
- Transportation-related accidents
- Urban air pollution
- Food contamination with pesticides
- Emerging and reemerging contagious infectious diseases
- Solid and hazardous waste accumulation
- Chemical and radiation hazards
- Deforestation and land degradation
- Climate change
- Ozone depletion
- Environmental or second-hand tobacco smoke

Modern hazards are linked with developed societies that lack the infrastructure and mechanisms to sustain development and protect the population's health and well-being.

The process by which societies move from traditional hazards to modern hazards is called risk transition (Landon, 2000; WHO, 1997). Modern, developed societies and developing societies must have well-designed developed and implemented mechanisms to ensure a healthy and safe risk transition. The first of these mechanisms involves the process of equitable, sustained development. As previously discussed, the Systems Model of Environmental Change can identify the multiaxial driving forces that threaten the health and well-being of populations. The second mechanism needed to ensure a safe, healthy risk transition is an adequate preventive population health enhancement program. Principles and practices of Public Health Management satisfy this endeavor and include the following programs:

- Immunization and chemoprophylaxis programs for all ages
- Potable water systems
- Communicable and contagious disease identification and treatment programs
- Sanitation engineering systems
- Preventive, age-specific, evidence-based health enhancement programs
- Age-specific, evidence-based health counseling

Those societies that can accomplish a successful risk transition and apply the mechanisms needed to maintain a safe, healthy population and environment will ensure a prosperous population growth politically, socially, and economically for both present and future generations.

ENVIRONMENTAL HEALTH RISK ASSESSMENT

To ensure the health and well-being for individuals and communities-at-large, a systematic process to assess the healthcare outcomes of people exposed to environmental agents must be in place. This systematic process of assessment is called an environmental health risk assessment (EHRA). This assessment is designed to measure the probabilities of how, when, where, and to what extent populations and their ecosystems may be affected by particular circumstances. It is also a process where data and information is gathered to characterize the potential healthcare outcomes of individuals and the community-at-large exposed to hazards, both traditional and modern, within their surrounding environment.

Risk, as previously defined, is the quantifiable measure of probability that given a specific set of circumstances—individuals, populations and ecosystems—will suffer disease, injury, death, or an adverse health-related outcome. Environmentally speaking, risk identifies the quantifiable measure of probability that the toxic properties of biological, chemical, and physical environmental agents will be produced in populations of individuals within their ecosystems under actual conditions of exposure (Rodricks, 1992).

Assessing environmental risk is an everyday activity. The measurement and perceptions of environmental risks are bound by a number of factors including but not limited to sociodemographics, culture, politics, and economics. Henceforth, it is inherently difficult to quantifiably measure the probability of environmental risk in populations of individuals. Adams (1995) proposed the following concept of risk compensation in order to better understand that the behavior of individuals within a population in any given situation, it is difficult to measure their environmental risk. Adams (1995) notes the following key observations about individual behavior:

- Everyone has the propensity to take risks.
- This propensity varies from individual to individual.
- This propensity is influenced by the potential rewards of risk taking.
- Perceptions of risk are influenced by the experience of accident losses (one's own and others).
- Individual risk taking decisions represent a balancing act in which perceptions of risk are weighed against the propensity to take risk.
- Accident losses are, by definition, a consequence of taking risks; the more risks an individual takes, the greater on average will be both for the rewards and losses he or she incurs.

It is evident from the model that Adams (1995) was trying to point out that individual behavior and possibly group behavior of the community-at-large is difficult to measure or quantify because of the uncertainties associated with individual behavior in general. Using Adams concept, one can begin to explore the question:

> What can affect the outcome of an
> environmental health risk assessment?

The outcome of an environmental health risk assessment may be affected by the following: individual or group behavior; the propensity for people to undertake risky behavior and the rewards and losses resulting from this behavior; the actions of other's behaviors; the nature of physical, chemical, and biological processes and the political, social, cultural, and economic issues within the community-at-large.

The primary objective for an EHRA is to quantify health risk behavior within the context of environmental exposures to biological, physical, and chemical agents within the ecosystem. The political, social, cultural, technical, and economic issues within the community-at-large directly and indirectly affects the healthcare outcomes management and planning of the population being evaluated. The main uses of EHRAs include appraising individual and population risks of specific exposures to biological, physical, and chemical agents in the ecosystem, estimating dose-response corresponding to a specific environmental risk, and quantifying environmental risk for regulatory, statutory, and administrative policy development at local, regional, national, and global venues (Landon, 2000).

There are several ways to quantify the outcome from an EHRA. In its simplest form, quantification can be categorized by severity or frequency of ill health experienced by the individual(s). For example, one can quantify severity of ill health to an exposure in the following manner:

- Mild injury or illness
- Moderate injury or illness
- Severe injury or illness requiring hospitalization
- Critical injury or illness requiring intensive medical/surgical care
- Death.

Obviously, this rudimentary quantification of exposure to an environmental agent does not provide a complete EHRA, and does not lead to understanding and improving healthcare outcomes management and planning from identified environmental exposures.

There is a well-recognized model for EHRAs that has been the accepted methodology since the 1970s (Paustenback, 2002). According to Paustenback (2002), many in the public health sector hope that EHRAs can bring order to the exponential growth and development of scientific and clinical data for potential health hazards and risks posed by biological, chemical, and physical agents in the environment. This accepted methodology has led to a systematic approach to EHRAs, thus producing sound administrative and clinical outcomes' analysis and decisions for improving the health and well-being of populations exposed to different environmental toxic agents.

According to Paustenback (2002), an EHRA is a "written document wherein all the pertinent scientific information, regarding toxicology, human experience, environmental fate, and exposure are assembled, critiqued, and interpreted." The goal of the EHRA is to estimate the probability of an adverse outcome on humans, wildlife, or ecosystems posed by a specific level of exposure to a biological, chemical, or physical hazard. Environmental HRAs are dependent on the degree of exposure to the hazard—the potency of the agent and the level of the exposure.

It is important to differentiate between the processes of environmental health risk assessment and environmental health risk management. In 1983, the National Academy of Science issued definitions for both processes (Paustenback, 2002). Environmental health risk assessment was to mean the following:

> The characterization of the potential adverse health effects of human exposures to environmental hazards. Risk assessments include several elements: description of the potential adverse health effects based on an evaluation of results of epidemiologic, clinical, toxicologic and environmental research, extrapolation from these results to predict the type and estimate the extent of health effects in humans under given conditions of exposure, judgments as to the number and characteristics of persons exposed at various intensities and durations, summary judgments on the existence and overall magnitude of the public-health problem, and characterization of the uncertainties inherent in the process of inferring risk.

Defining the term "environmental health risk management," the National Academy of Science report used the following definition:

> The process of evaluating alternative regulatory actions and selecting among them. Risk management which is carried out by regulatory agencies under various legislative mandates is an agency decision-making process that entails consideration of political, social, economic, and engineering information with risk-related information to develop, analyze, and compare regulatory options and to select the appropriate regulatory response to a potential chronic health hazard. The selection process necessarily

requires the use of value judgments on such issues as the acceptability of risk and the reasonableness of the costs of control.

Clearly, the separation of environmental health risk assessment from environmental health risk management is important to remove as much bias from the scientific methodology and the action plans of agencies developed from the data presented by the scientists and clinicians at the point of care. The classic model of EHRA is divided into four distinct steps including: hazard identification, dose-response assessment, exposure assessment, and risk characterization.

Hazard identification is the most easily recognized step of the assessment process. This step must always begin the assessment; it is the process of determining whether human exposure to a biological, chemical, or physical agent could cause an increase in the incidence of a health condition (e.g., cancer, birth defect, etc.) or whether exposure of a nonhuman receptor (e.g., wildlife, fish, fowl, etc.) might be adversely affected. Hazard identification involves characterizing the nature and strength of the evidence of causation. Unfortunately, there are only a few biological, chemical, or physical agents for which human data definitively links a cause and adverse effect, such as cancer (i.e., presumptive diagnosis). Extrapolation from laboratory animal studies in which a direct cause and effect can be established serves as evidence that an agent may cause cancer for any exposed human.

Dose-response assessment, the second step of the EHRA, is the process of characterizing the relationship between the amount or dose of an agent administered or received and the incidence of an adverse health effect in exposed populations. Dose-response assessment also estimates the incidence of the effect as a function of exposure to the biological, physical, or chemical agent. This step considers the following factors as part of the dose-response assessment: intensity of exposure, age pattern of exposure, sociodemographic variables, and individual lifestyle behavior. A dose-response assessment often requires extrapolation from high to low doses and extrapolation from animals to humans, or one laboratory animal species to a species of wildlife. A dose-response assessment should describe and justify the methods of extrapolation used to predict incidence, and it should characterize the statistical and biological uncertainties of the scientific and clinical methodology in a quantifiable manner.

The third step, exposure assessment, is the process of estimating the intensity, frequency, and duration of human or animal exposure to a biological, physical, or chemical agent currently present in the environment, or of estimating hypothetical exposures that may potentially arise from the release of new agents into the environment. The exposure assessment must be as complete as possible and the assessment should include the following: description of the amount, duration, schedule and route of exposure (e.g., ingestion, inhalation, dermal absorption), the size, nature, and classes of the human, animal, aquatic, or wildlife populations exposed, and the quantifiable uncertainties in all the estimates of exposure. The exposure assessment is often used to identify, design, develop, and implement prospective environmental control procedures as well as to predict the health outcomes of available control technologies that may limit environmental exposure.

The fourth and final step of the EHRA is risk characterization. Risk characterization is the process of estimating the incidence of a health effect under the various conditions of human or animal exposure described in the exposure assessment. Risk characterization is performed by combining the exposure and dose-response assessment. The summary effects of the quantifiable and qualitative uncertainties noted in the three previous steps of the EHRA are described and discussed in great detail as part of the risk characterization step.

The quantitative estimate of risk, the size of exposed population, and the uncertainty surrounding the risks estimates (i.e., risk characterization) are the topics of principal interest to those managing environmental risk. The private, industrial, or agricultural corporation or the public agencies responsible for managing environmental health risk must consider the results of the risk characterization when evaluating the economics, societal effects, and various benefits of the EHRA. Factors such as societal norms, cultural differences, technological uncertainties, cost-benefit relationships, cost-effectiveness, and severity of the identified potential hazards and risks to the population influence how decision makers, both public and private, respond to EHRAs. The more informed the decision makers are the better the health-care outcomes management and planning for the exposed population at risk.

RISK MANAGEMENT

The definition of health risk management is following the principles, criteria, or prevailing techniques used to identify, investigate, analyze, evaluate, and select the most advantageous methods reducing, modifying, correcting, or eliminating identifiable risks (Florida Administrative Code,

Dept of Insurance). The purpose of managing risk is to avoid or reduce losses of resources and minimize the effects of losses on a business through careful planning, organization, and administration. Losses may result from events such as natural disaster, lawsuits, personnel turnover, business interruption, and changes in governmental policy. A single loss may affect various areas of individual interest including property, personal injury, net income, and liability.

The evolution of risk management arose out of response to the growing medical malpractice litigation that peaked in the 1980s. Consumer expectations have changed significantly; patients increasingly seek complex life-prolonging medical procedures (e.g., organ transplantation, heart bypass surgery, angioplasty, dental implants). Patients remain uneducated that complex treatments often bear increased outcome risks in spite of signing informed consent forms, and maintain inflated expectations, demanding perfection from the healthcare delivery system and clinicians. Healthcare providers have become the scapegoats for adverse patient outcomes and juries tend to be sympathetic to those who experience even blameless tragedy.

The risk manager has evolved over time as a result of increased litigation in all healthcare venues. The duties of the risk include:

- Legal
- Patient care ombudsman
- Operations
- Staff function supports line operations
- Regulatory/statutory compliance
- Risk aversion
- Standards of care
- Employee training
- Incident/accident investigation

The need for risk management and the risk manager is a direct result of increasing professional requirements, insurance restrictions, legal threats, and changes in healthcare delivery. These changes include new laws, regulations, and rules; medical advances in patient care; threat of current and emerging chronic disease states; growing public demand for accountability in health care; evolution of managed care delivery systems; and healthcare service reduction and loss of choice by patients seeking high quality and easily accessible clinical care. The public demand for accountability has focused on protecting the public, protecting the environment, exposing fraud and unsafe medical practices, and extending and preserving the individual rights of patients. The reduction in healthcare delivery services has occurred as a direct result of professional staffing reductions in hospitals (e.g., registered and licensed practical nurses), administrative position elimination, redefining patient/nurse ratio, reductions in employee benefits and compensation and the cross-training of lower level professional (i.e., medical assistants) personnel.

The goals of risk management with respects to healthcare outcomes management and planning include the following: identifying exposure to loss by categorizing losses unique to the situation, analyzing loss exposure with respects to the cost significance in each exposure category—to preventing loss and repairing damages, assessing alternative risk management techniques with strategies available to prevent, minimize, or control the exposure, selecting the best method to control the loss, and implementing a well-defined risk management program with objectives that are measurable to determine the success of the program.

There are many factors that affect the perception of risk by individuals and populations including familiarity, control, proximity in space and time, the dread factor, and the scale factor. If the risk is unfamiliar to an individual or if he/she perceives that he/she does not have control of the situation, the perceived risk will be high and individuals will require stronger protection by both the private corporations and public agencies. Being closer to risk in terms of physical space increases the perception of risk by individuals as well. In terms of time, immediacy (that is the newness of the risk such as a nuclear reactor that has just been built and is going on line for the first time or a new radiologic procedure that has just been approved for general use) can increase the perception of risk. The dread factor is high when catastrophe is perceived to imminent. Finally, the scale factor is perceived to be high when a large number of individuals or the community-at-large may be injured or killed because of potential exposure to a particular hazard and risk. In general, perception of risk can be graded as high, medium, or low.

The effective communication of risk is critical to lowering the perception of risk by individuals and the community-at-large. Effective risk communication by the risk manager or an appropriate person should have the following characteristics:

- Accept and involve the public as a legitimate partner
- Plan carefully and evaluate the process

- Listen to the public's specific concerns
- Be honest, frank, and open
- Coordinate and collaborate with other credible sources
- Meet the needs of the media
- Speak clearly and with compassion

Increasingly, health constituencies (see Table 1-1) are expressing a need to have the implications for the quality of life (a healthcare outcome) recognized alongside the quantitative assessments of risk (Landon, 2000). Criteria for assessing the quality of life with respects to risk management may include aesthetics (visual impact, noise, and smell), economic well-being (loss of job), fairness (inequity of costs and benefits to individual), future generations (inequity of costs' burdens), health and well-being (morbidity and mortality), peace of mind (the dread and scale factor), recreation, and sense of community.

Many countries, including the United States, have statutory and regulatory requirements for new projects that may have an effect on the health and well-being of the population. For example, when building a new healthcare facility or when bringing in new healthcare technology, an environmental impact assessment would be done (Gilpin, 1995). The environmental impact assessment should consider the effects on the population from an ecological and biological perspective (i.e., pollution, climate change, etc.), natural resources, and psychosocial and economic effects on the population.

Risk management is concerned with implementing decisions about tolerating or changing risk to public health (Landon, 2000). Risk management is often carried out by governmental agencies. However, the private sector, especially healthcare delivery systems, has become increasingly concerned about mitigating exposure as a result of changing healthcare consumer expectations. Part of the strategy for risk management is to consider the risk assessment within a wider context—using a biopsychosocial approach along with political and economic considerations. Engineering controls, the ability to limit or control a particular hazard or risk to individuals and the community-at-large, and the limits of detection of biological, chemical, and physical agents may improve the overall safety to the public and improve the health and well-being resulting in acceptable healthcare outcomes. Weighing the acceptability of the risk and the cost of controlling exposures is the main objective of the risk manager. There are a multitude of frameworks used by risk managers that are based on available scientific as well as clinical data and information on the nature of the risk. The tolerability of the risk to the general population is really an estimation of constraints (i.e., setting dose limits above which persons should not be normally exposed) and optimization (i.e., the balancing of the costs and benefits of proposed risk reduction measures). Finally, understanding how all health constituencies perceive risks is very important to the effective communication and management of risk.

CONCLUSION

Understanding environmental health issues is another factor in improving healthcare outcomes management and planning. Environmental health management requires a biopsychosocial approach to identifying health risks and then applying a multidimensional plan to improve the health and well-being of those affected by the risk. More needs to be done in healthcare delivery to quantify environmental health hazards and risks and incorporate this information into the overall healthcare interventions to improve population and individual healthcare outcomes.

References

1. Abramson, JH. *Survey methods in community medicine*. Edinburgh: Churchill Livingston; 1990.
2. Acheson, D. *Tackling inequalities in health*. London, England: The King's Fund; 1995.
3. Adams, MR, Moss, MO. *Food microbiology*. London, England: Royal Society of Chemistry; 1995.
4. Akabas, SH, Galvin, DE. *Disability management: A complete system to reduce costs, increase productivity, meet employee needs, and ensure legal compliance*. New York, NY: American Medical Association Communications; 1992.
5. Altman, DG. Strategies for community health intervention: Promise, paradoxes, pitfalls. *Psychol Med* 1995; 57:226–233.
6. American Medical Association. *Guides to the evaluation of permanent impairment*. 5th edition. Chicago, IL: American Medical Association Press; 2000.
7. American Medical Association. *Roadmaps for clinical practice: A primer on population-based medicine*. Chicago, IL: American Medical Association; 2002.
8. Americans with Disabilities Act, HR Rep No. 101-485, pt3, at 23 (1990), reprinted in 1990 USCCN 445, 446.
9. Association of American Medical Colleges. *Contemporary issues in medicine: Medical informatics and population health; Medical school objectives project report II*. June, 1998.

10. *Backgrounder on demand management.* The Change Foundation for the Demand Management Think Tank, Boulevard Club, Toronto, Ontario, January 23, 2002. www.changefoundation.com.

11. Balas, EA, Boros, SA. Managing clinical knowledge for health care improvement. *Yearbook of Medical Informatics* 2000; 65–70.

12. Beauchamp, T, Childress, J. *Principles of biomedical ethics,* 4th edition. Oxford, England: Oxford University Press; 1994.

13. Bechman, HB, Markakis, KM, Suchman, AL, Frankel, RM. The doctor-patient relationship and malpractice: Lessons from plaintiff depositions. *Arch Int Med* 1994; 154:1365–1370.

14. Beery, WL, Schoenback, VJ, Wagner, EH et al. *Health risk appraisal: Methods and programs with annotated bibliography.* Washington, DC: National Center for Health Services Research and Health Care Technology; 1986.

15. Berwick, DM, Godfrey, AB, Roessner, J. *Curing health care: New strategies for quality improvement.* San Francisco, CA: Jossey-Bass Publishers, Inc.; 1990.

16. Blane, D. The life course, the social gradient and health. In: Marmot, M and Wilkinson, R, eds. *Social determinants of health.* New York, NY: Oxford University Press; 1999, 64–80.

17. Brandt, EN, Pope, AM. *Enabling America: Assessing the role of rehabilitation science and engineering.* Washington, DC: National Academy Press; 1997.

18. Brown, MM, Brown, GC, Sharma, S. *Evidence-based to value-based medicine.* Chicago, IL: AMA Press; 2005.

19. Bruyere, S. *Disability employment policies and practices in private and federal sector organizations.* Ithaca, NY: Cornell University; 2000.

20. Burkhauser, RV, Butler, JS, Kim, YM. The importance of employer accommodation on the job duration of workers with disabilities: A hazard model approach. *Labour Economics* 1995; 2(2):109–130.

21. Butler, RJ, Gardner, BD, Gardner, HH. More than cost shifting: Moral hazard lowers productivity. *The Journal of Risk and Insurance* 1998; 65(4):671–688.

22. Cassel, EJ. The nature of suffering and the goals of medicine. *New England Journal of Medicine* 1982; 306:639–645.

23. Centers for Disease Control and Prevention. Prevalence of healthy lifestyle characteristics—Michigan, 1998–2000. *MMWR* 2001; 50:758–761.

24. Centers for Disease Control and Prevention. *Measuring healthy days.* Atlanta, GA: CDC; 2000.

25. CMS, office of the Actuary, 2002.

26. Centers for Medicare and Medicaid Services. Office of the Actuary at the Centers for Medicare and Medicaid Services. National healthcare expenditures projections: 2001–2011. Available at www.cms.hhs.gov. Accessed June 30, 2005.

27. Centers for Medicare and Medicaid Services. National healthcare expenditures aggregate and per capita amounts, percent distribution, and average annual percent growth, by source of funds: selected calendar years 1960–1999. Available at www.cms.hhs.gov. Accessed June 30, 2005.

28. Chassin, MR, Galvin, RW. The urgent need to improve health care quality. *Journal of the American Medical Association* 1998; 280(11):1000–1005.

29. Cochrane, AL. *Effectiveness and efficiency*. London: Nuffield Provincial Hospitals Trust; 1972.

30. Cockerham, WC. *Medical Sociology*. 9th edition. Upper Saddle River, NJ: Pearson/Prentice Hall; 2004.

31. Cohen, JA. A coefficient of agreement for nominal scales. *Educ Psychol Meas* 1960; 20:37–46.

32. Coyne, JC, Fechner-Bates, S, Schwenk, TL. Prevalence, nature and comorbidity of depressive disorders in primary care. *General Hospital Psychiatry* 1994; 16:267–276.

33. Danczyk-Hawley, CE, McMahon, BT, Flynn, BG. Progression of disability benefits as a measure of disability management program effectiveness: implications for future research. In: McMahon, BT, Kregal, J, Wehman, P. eds. *An evaluation of the progression of disability benefits among workers in American industry: impact, outcomes and implications*. Virginia Commonwealth University Press, Richmond, VA. 2000, http://www.worksupport.com/main/downloads/podchap5.pdf.

34. Defriese, GH, Fielding, JE. Health risk appraisal in the 1990's: Opportunities, challenges, and expectations. *Annu Rev Public Health* 1990; 11:401–418.

35. Demers, R, Neale, A, Adams, R, Trembath, C, Herman, S. The impact of physicians' brief smoking cessation counseling: A MIRNET study. *J Fam Pract* 1990; 31:625–629.

36. Dever, GA. *Improving outcomes in public health practice: Strategy and methods*. Gaithersburg, MD: Aspen Publishers; 1997.

37. Deyo, R, Diehl, A. Patient satisfaction with medical care for low back pain. *Spine* 1986; 11:28–30.

38. Donabedian, A. *An introduction to quality assurance in health care*. New York, NY: Oxford University Press, Inc.; 2003.

39. Donabedian, A. Measuring health. "Evaluational uses of measures of morbidity and health," In: *Aspects of medical care administration: Specifying requirements for health care*. Cambridge, MA: Harvard University Press, Inc.; 1973.

40. Donabedian, A. *The criteria and standards of quality*. Volume II of *Explorations in quality assessment and monitoring*. Ann Arbor, MI: Health Administration Press, Inc.; 1982.

41. Donabedian, A. The role of outcomes in quality assessment and assurance. *Quality Review Bulletin* 1986; 18:356–360.

42. Donelan, K, Blendon, RJ, Schoen, C, Davis, K, Binns, K. The cost of health system change: Public discontent in five nations. *Health Affairs* 1999; 18(3):206–216.

43. Dowrick, CF. Rethinking the doctor-patient relationship in general practice. *Health Soc Care Commun* 1997; 5:11–14.

44. Drummond, ME, O'Brien, B, Stoddart, GL, Torrence, GW. *Methods for the economic evaluation of health care programmes*. 2nd edition. New York, NY: Oxford University Press; 1999.

45. Dubos, R. *The mirage of health.* New York, NY: Harper and Row; 1959.
46. Eisenberg, JM. Quality research for quality healthcare: The data connection. *Health Services Research* 2000; 35:XII–XVII.
47. Engel, GL. The need for a new medical model: A challenge for biomedicine. *Science* 1977; 196:129–136.
48. Engel, GL. The clinical application of the biopsychosocial model. *American Journal of Psychiatry* 1980; 137:5.
49. Engel, GL. How much longer must medicine's science be bounded by seventeenth century world view? *The task of medicine: Dialogue at Wickenburg.* Menlo Park, CA: The Henry Kaiser Family Foundation; 1988: 113–126.
50. Epstein, RM, Morse, DS, Williams, GC, leRoux, P, Suchman, AL, Quill, TE. Clinical practice and the biopsychosocial approach. In: Frankel, RM, Quill, TE, McDaniel, SH, eds. *The biopsychosocial approach: Past, present, and future.* Rochester, NY: University of Rochester Press; 2003: 33–66.
51. Epstein, RM. The patient-physician relationship. In: Mengel, MB, Holleman, WL, eds. *Fundamentals of Clinical Practice: A textbook on the patient, doctor and society.* New York, NY: Plenum Medical Book Company; 1996:105–132.
52. Epstein, RS, Sherwood, LM. From outcomes research to disease management: A guide for the perplexed. *Ann Int Med* 1996; 124(9):832–837.
53. Escobar, JI. Overview of somatization: Diagnosis, epidemiology, and management. *Psychopharmacology Bulletin* 1996; 32:589–596.
54. Feigenbaum, AV. *Total quality control.* 1st edition. New York, NY: McGraw Hill; 1951.
55. Fitzpatrick, R. The assessment of patient satisfaction. In: Jenkinson, C. ed. *Assessment and evaluation of health and medical care: A methods text.* Buckingham, England: Open University Press; 1997:XXX.
56. Fitzpatrick, R, Boulton, M. Qualitative methods for assessing health care. *Quality in Health Care* 1994; 3:107–113.
57. Fitzpatrick, R, Hopkins, A. Patients' satisfaction with communication in neurological outpatient clinics. *Journal of Psychosomatic Research* 1981; 25:329–334.
58. Flexner, A. *Medical education in the United States and Canada.* New York, NY: Carnegie Foundation for the Advancement of Teaching; 1910.
59. Florida Administrative Code, Chapter 4-217, Dept of Insurance.
60. Flynn, B. *Best practices of organizations utilizing disability management strategies.* 2000.
61. Frame, PS. Health maintenance in clinical practice: Strategies and barriers. *American Family Physician* 1992; 3:1192–1200.
62. Frankel, RM, Quill, TE, McDaniel, SH. *The biopsychosocial approach: Past, present, and future.* Rochester, NY: University of Rochester Press; 2003.
63. Freitas, R. Doubling of medical knowledge. Available at: http://discussforesight.org/critmail/sci_nano/5165/html. Accessed June 30, 2005.
64. Friedman, GD. *Primer of Epidemiology.* 5th edition. New York, NY: The McGraw-Hill Companies, Inc.; 2004.

65. Froom, P. Benbassat, J. Inconsistencies in the classification of preventive interventions. *Prev Med* 2000; 31:153–158.

66. Galvin, DE. Health promotion, disability management, and rehabilitation in the workplace. *Rehabilitation Literature* 1986; 47(9–10):218–223.

67. Gilpin, A. *Environmental impact assessment: Cutting edge for the 21st century.* Cambridge, MA: Cambridge University Press; 1995.

68. Gold, MR, Siegel, JE, Russell, LB, Weinstein, MC, eds. *Cost-effectiveness in health and medicine.* New York, NY: Oxford University Press; 1996.

69. Gordon, M, Rehm, S. *Vital signs: Taking the pulse of your practice. Volume 1. Patient satisfaction surveys.* Kansas City, MO: American Academy of Family Physicians; 1996.

70. Harper, AC, Lambert, LJ. *The health of populations: An introduction.* 2nd edition. New York, NY: Springer Publishing Company; 1994.

71. Herzlinger, RE. The failed revolution in health care—The role of management. *Harvard Business Review* 1989; 67(2):95–106.

72. Higgins, M, Enright, P, Kronmal, R, Schenker, M, Anton-Culver, H, Lyles, M. Smoking and lung function in elderly men and women: The cardiovascular health study. *Journal of the American Medical Association* 1993; 269:2741–2748.

73. Hoffman, C, Rice, DP, Sung, HY. Persons with chronic conditions. Their prevalence and costs. *Journal of the American Medical Association* 1996; 276(18):1473–1479.

74. Hull, D. Reduction and genetics. *Journal of Medicine and Philosophy* 1981; 6.

75. Institute of Medicine. *To err is human: Building a safer health system.* Washington, DC: National Academy Press; 2000.

76. Institute of Medicine. *Crossing the quality chasm: A new health system for the 21st century.* Washington, DC: National Academy Press; 2001.

77. Jarviskowski, J, Lahelma, E. *Early rehabilitation at the workplace.* New York, NY: World Rehabilitation Fund; 1980.

78. Jekel, JF, Elmore, JG, Katz, DL. *Epidemiology, biostatistics, and preventive medicine.* Philadelphia, PA: WB Saunders Company; 1996.

79. Jenkinson, C. *Assessment and evaluation of health and medical care: A methods text.* Buckingham, England: Open University Press; 1997.

80. Kant, I. *The critique of practical reason.* New York, NY: Macmillan; 1985.

81. Kass, L. *Toward a more natural science: Biology and human affairs.* New York, NY: The Free Press; 1985.

82. Klarman, H, Francis, J, Rosenthal, G. Cost-effectiveness applied to the treatment of chronic renal disease. *Medical Care* 1968; 6:48–55.

83. Krueger, RA. *Focus groups. A practical guide for applied research.* Thousand Oaks, CA: Sage; 1994.

84. Kuby, M, Harner, J, Gober, P. *Human geography in action.* New York, NY: John Wiley and Sons; 1998.

85. Kuhn, TS. *The structure of scientific revolutions.* Chicago, IL: The University of Chicago Press; 1962.

86. Landon, M. Health and the environment. In: *Environmental health, health systems management study unit 306.* London, England: London School of Hygiene and Tropical Medicine; 2000.

87. Layte, R, Jenkinson, C. Social surveys. In: Jenkinson, C. ed. *Assessment and evaluation of health and medical care: A methods text.* Buckingham, England: Open University Press; 1997.

88. Lee, K, Mill, A. The economics of health in developing countries: A critical review. In: Lee, K and Mill, A., eds. *The economics of health in developing countries.* New York, NY: Oxford University Press; 1983.

89. Leplege, A, Hunt, S. The problem of quality of life in medicine. *Journal of the American Medical Association* 1997; 278:47–50.

90. Lin, EH, Katon, W, Von Korff, M, et al. Frustrating patients: Physician and patient perspectives among distressed high users of medical services. *J Gen Int Medicine* 1991; 6:241–246.

91. Lipkin, M, Lybrand, WA, eds. *Population-based medicine.* New York, NY: Praeger Publishers; 1982.

92. Lohr, KN. *Medicare: A strategy for quality assurance.* Washington, DC: National Academy Press; 1990.

93. Longino, CF, Murphy, JW. *The old age challenge to the biomedical model: Paradigm strain and health policy.* Amityville, NY: Baywood Publishing Company, Inc.; 1995.

94. Mark, A, Pencheon, D, Elliott, R. Demanding healthcare. *International Journal of Health Planning and Management* 2000; 15:237–253.

95. Marks, DF, Murray, M, Evans, B, Willig, C. *Health psychology: Theory, research and practice.* London, England: Sage Publications; 2000.

96. Maxwell, R. Quality assessment in health. *British Medical Journal* 1984; 288:1470–1472.

97. McGinnis, JM, Foege, W. Actual causes of death in the United States. *Journal of the American Medical Association* 1993; 270:2207–2212.

98. McMahon, BT, Danczyk-Hawley, CE, Reid, CA, Habeck, R, Kregal, J, Owens, P. Progression of disability benefits. In: McMahon, BT, Kregal, J, Wehman, P. eds. *An evaluation of the progression of disability benefits among workers in American industry: Impact, outcomes and implications.* Richmond, VA: Virginia Commonwealth University Press; 2000. Available at: http://www.worksupport.com/main/downloads/podchap1.pdf.

99. McMichael, AJ. *Planet overload: Global environmental change and the health of the human species.* Cambridge, MA: University Press; 1993.

100. McNeil, P. *Research methods.* London, England: Routledge; 1990.

101. Mills, A, Gilson, L. *Health economics for developing countries: A survival kit.* London, England: London School of Hygiene and Tropical Medicine; 1988.

102. Milsum, JH. Lifestyle changes for the whole person: Stimulation through health hazard appraisal. In: Davidson, PO, Davidson, SM. eds. *Behavioral Medicine.* New York, NY: Brunner Mazel; 1980:116–150.

103. Mooney, GH. Equity in health care: Confronting the confusion. *Effective Health Care* 1983; 1:179–194.

104. Moore, CM. *Group techniques for idea building.* Thousand Oaks, CA: Sage; 1994.

105. National Research Council. *Networking health: Prescriptions for the Internet.* Washington, DC: National Academy Press; 2000.

106. Neese, RE, Hagedorn, SD, Scheitel, SM, et al. Disease management strategies: Managing care giving in managed care. *Quality Mgmt in Health Care* 2000; 9(1):42–48.

107. Oster, G, Thompson, D, Edelsberg, J, Bird, A, Colditz, G. Lifetime health and economic benefits of weight loss among obese persons. *American Journal of Public Health* 1999; 89:1539–1542.

108. Patrick, DL, Deyo, RA. Generic and disease-specific measures in assessing health status and quality of life. *Medical Care* 1989; 27(3):S217–S232.

109. Paustenback, DJ. Primer on human and environmental risk assessment. In: Paustenback, DJ eds. *Human and ecological risk assessment: Theory and practice.* New York, NY: Wiley and Sons, Inc.; 2002.

110. Pencheon, D. Matching demand and supply fairly and efficiently. *British Medical Journal* 1998; 316:1665–1667.

111. Petty, T. It's never too late to stop smoking: But how old are your lungs? *Journal of the American Medical Association* 1993; 269:2785–2786.

112. Powell, DR. Implementing a medical self-care program. *Employee Benefits Journal* 2003; 28(3):40–42.

113. Powell, DR. The *health, economic, and legal implications of medical self-care programs.* Farmington Hills, MI: American Institute of Preventive Medicine; 2001.

114. Rafuse, J. Evidence-based medicine means MDs must develop new skills, attitudes: CMA conference told. *Can Med Assoc J* 1994; 150:1479–1481.

115. Rawls, J. *A theory of justice.* Cambridge, MA: Harvard University Press; 1971.

116. Ray, G, Thomas, TL, Fireman, B, et al. The cost of health conditions in a health maintenance organization. *Medical Care Res and Rev* 2000; 57(1):92–109.

117. Reno, VP, Mashow, JL, Gradison, B, eds. *Disability: Challenges for social insurance, health care financing, and labor market policy.* Washington, DC: National Academy of Social Insurance; 1997.

118. Robbins, L, Hall, J. *How to practice prospective medicine.* Indianapolis, IN: Methodist Hospital of Indiana; 1970.

119. The Robert Wood Johnson Foundation. *Chronic care in America: A 21st century challenge.* Princeton, NJ: The Robert Wood Johnson Foundation; 1996.

120. Rodricks, JV. *Calculated risks: The toxicity and human health risks of chemicals in our environment.* Cambridge, MA: University Press; 1992.

121. Rogers, A, Entwistle, V, Pencheon, D. A patient led HNS: Managing demand at the interface between lay and primary care. *British Medical Journal* 1998; 316:1816–1819.

122. Ross, JL. Work programs lag in promoting return to work. Testimony before the Special Subcommittee on Aging, US Senate. *GAO/T-EHS-96-147.* 1996; 6.

123. Rothman, SS. *Lessons from the living cell: The limits of reductionism.* New York, NY: McGraw-Hill; 2002.

124. Rupp, K, Stapleton, DC. eds. *Growth in disability benefits: Explanations and policy implications.* Kalamazoo, MI: Upjohn Institute for Employment Research; 1998.

125. Schoenback, VJ, Wagner, EH, Beery, WL. Health risk appraisal: Review of evidence for effectiveness. *Health Services Research* 1987; 22(4):553–580.

126. Schuster, MA, McGlynn, EA, Brook, RH. How good is the quality of health care in the United States? *Milbank Quarterly* 1998; 76:517–563.

127. Schwartz, G. Disability costs: The impending crisis. *Business and Health.* 1984; 5.

128. Shrey, DE, Lacerte, M. *Principles and practice of disability management in industry.* Winter Park, FL: GR Press, Inc.; 1995.

129. Sinclair, J, Torrence GW, Boyle, M, Horwood, M, Saigal, S, Sackett, D. Evaluation of neonatal intensive care programs. *New England Journal of Medicine* 1981; 305:489–494.

130. Sinclair, D. Measuring humanity. In *Health Care Evaluation, Health Systems Management Study Unit 204.* London, England: London School of Hygiene and Tropical Medicine; 2000.

131. Stewart, M, Brown, JB, Donner, A, et al. The impact of patient-centered care on patient's outcomes. *Journal of Family Practice* 2000; 49:796–804.

132. Stewart, M, Brown, JB, Donner, A, et al. *Final report: The impact of patient-centered care on patient outcomes in Family Practice.* Grant 1046; London, England: University of Western Ontario; 1997.

133. Stone, DH. Design a questionnaire. *British Medical Journal* 1993; 307: 1264–1266.

134. *Sutton v United Airlines.* 1999; 97 US 1943.

135. Tengs, TO, Adams, ME, Pliskin, JP, et al. Five hundred life-saving interventions and their cost-effectiveness. *Risk Analysis* 1995; 15:369–390.

136. Thomas, JW, Longo, DR. Applications of severity measurement systems for hospital quality management. *Hospital and Health Administration* 1990; 35: 221–243.

137. Torrence, GW, Siegel, JE, Luce, BR. Framing and designing the cost-effectiveness analysis. In: Gold, MR, Siegel, JE, Russell, LB, Weinstein, MC, eds. *Cost-effectiveness in health and medicine.* New York, NY: Oxford University Press; 1996.

138. United States General Accounting Office: Social Security disability insurance: Multiple factors affect beneficiaries' ability to return to work. Report to the chairman, subcommittee on Social Security, Committee on Ways and Means, House of Representatives. *GAO/HEHS-98-39* 1998.

139. Van Gaal, L, Waunters, M, De Leeuw, I. The beneficial effects of modest weight loss on cardiovascular risk factors. *Int J Obes Rel Metab Disord* 1997; 21:S5–S9.

140. Vickery, DM, Lynch, WD. Demand management: Enabling patients to use medical care appropriately. *JOEM* 1995; 37:551–557.

141. Wadsworth, M. Early life. In: Marmot, M and Wilkinson, R, eds. *Social Determinants of Health.* New York, NY: Oxford University Press; 1999, 44–63.

142. Wagner, EH, Austin, BT, Von Korff, M. Organizing care for patients with chronic illness. *Milbank Quarterly* 1996; 74(4):511–544.

143. Wagner, EH. Managed care and chronic illness: Health services research needs. *Health Serv Res* 1997; 32:702–714.

144. Ware, JE, Sherbourne, CD. The MOS 36 item short-form health survey (SF-36) conceptual framework and item selection. *Medical Care* 1992; 30:473–483.

145. Watson Wyatt/WGBH. *Staying at work: Increasing shareholder value through integrated disability management, third annual survey.* Washington, DC: Watson Wyatt; 1999.

146. Watson Wyatt/WGBH. *Staying at work: Improving health and productivity. Fifth annual Watson Wyatt/WGBH survey on integrated disability management.* Washington, DC: Watson Wyatt; 2000.

147. Wee, C, McCarthy, E, Davis, R, Phillips, R. Physician counseling about exercise. *Journal of the American Medical Association* 1999; 228:1583–1588.

148. Weinstein, MC, Stasson, WB. Foundation of cost-effective analysis for health and medical practice. *New England Journal of Medicine* 1977; 296:716–721.

149. Weiss, B, Senf, J. Patient satisfaction survey instrument for use in health maintenance organizations. *Medical Care* 1990; 28:434–445.

150. Wennberg, JE. Improving the medical decision making process. *Health Affairs* 1988; 7(1):99–106.

151. Wheeler, DJ, Chambers, DS. *Understanding Statistical Process Control.* 2nd edition. Knoxville, TN: SPC Press; 1992.

152. White, KL, Williams, TF, Greenberg, BG. The ecology of medical care. *New England Journal of Medicine* 1961; 265:885–892.

153. Williamson, D. Intentional weight loss: Patterns in the general population and its association with morbidity and mortality. *Int J Obes Rel Metab Disord* 1997; 21:S14–S19.

154. Wilson, IB, Cleary, PD. Linking clinical variables with health-related quality of life: A conceptual model of patient outcomes. *Journal of the American Medical Association* 1995; 273:59–65.

155. Woodruff, CB, Carney, P, Dietrich, AJ. *Cancer prevention in community practice: Office systems workbook.* Hanover, NH: Trustees of Dartmouth College; 1992.

156. World Health Organization. *Preamble to the Constitution of the World Health Organization as adopted by the International Health Conference.* New York, NY: June 19–22, 1946; signed on 22 July 1946 by the representatives of 61 States (Official Records of the World Health Organization, no. 2, p. 100) and entered into force on April 7, 1948.

157. World Health Organization. *Our planet, our health: Report of the WHO commission on health and environment.* Geneva, Switzerland: WHO; 1992.

158. World Health Organization. *Global strategy: Health, environment and development: Approaches to drafting country-wide strategies for human well-being under Agenda 21.* Geneva, Switzerland: WHO; 1993.

159. World Health Organization. *Health and environment in sustainable development: Five years after the Earth Summit.* Geneva, Switzerland: WHO; 1997.

160. World Medical Organization. Declaration of Helsinki. *British Medical Journal* 1996; 313(7070):1448–1449.

161. Zanner, R. *Ethics and the clinical encounter.* Englewood Cliffs, NJ: Prentice Hall; 1988.

162. Ziebland, S, Wright, L. Qualitative research methods. In: Jenkinson, C., ed. *Assessment and evaluation of health and medical care: A methods text.* Buckingham, England: Open University Press; 1997.

163. Zucker, A. Holism and reductionism: A view from genetics. *Journal of Medicine and Philosophy* 1981; 6.

INDEX

Page numbers followed by t denote tables